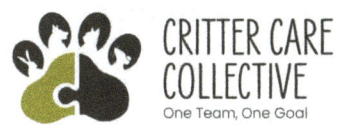

THE DOG OWNER'S GUIDE TO HEALTH EMERGENCIES

Essential Tips to Recognize, Respond, and Prepare for Dog Emergencies

Written by:

Dr. Gal Chivvis

Emergency Veterinarian

To my family and friends who cheered me on and provided support through this adventure!
Thank you!!!
~GC

Copyright © 2025 Critter Care Collective, LLC

All rights reserved. No part of this publication may be reproduced, distributed, or transmitted in any form or by any means, including photocopying, recording, or other electronic or mechanical methods, without the prior written permission of the publisher, except in the case of brief quotations embodied in critical reviews or certain other noncommercial uses permitted by copyright law. For permission requests, email the publisher, with "Attention: Permissions Coordinator" in the subject line to the following email: crittercarecollective@gmail.com.

Printed by Kindle Direct Publishing
ISBN: 979-8-9920483-8-4 (paperback)
ISBN: 979-8-9920483-9-1 (Kindle Ebook)

Written by Dr. Gal Chivvis, DVM
Cover and interior design by Dr. Gal Chivvis and Wendy Reed
Editor: Tina Wismer, DVM, MS, DABVT, DABT

First printing, 2025

Business Address:
5000 Thayer Center
STE C
Oakland, MD 21550

Printed in the United States of America

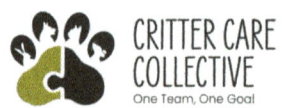

MY DOG'S NAME:

_____

My local veterinarian's name, phone number, and address:

_____
_____
_____

Emergency veterinarian contact information:

_____
_____
_____

ASPCA POISON CONTROL
(888) 426-4435

A Note to Dog Families

As a loving pet owner, your primary goal is to ensure your dog remains happy and healthy. However, emergencies can arise unexpectedly and knowing when to act quickly can be crucial to ensuring your pup's wellbeing - and can even save your dog's life. In this book, I'll help you discern between minor issues and genuine emergencies, and I'll highlight the warning signs that necessitate immediate attention.

Keep in mind that these are general guidelines only. Sometimes emergencies can be difficult to spot and don't fit the classic signs. Ultimately, YOU know your pup best, so if you have concerns - please reach out to a veterinarian.

Before we begin, let's get some things out of the way.

DISCLAIMER
I created this book to provide a source of education for pet owners because I believe we achieve the best possible care for our pets when pet families and veterinary members work together as a team!

The information included within this text is from my personal experience as an emergency veterinarian. It is intended to provide guidance/education but is in no way intended to provide a diagnosis or replace the need to seek care for your pet. Be advised that all vets do things a little differently. So, my approach to the situations described may differ from that of your veterinarian. ALWAYS follow the recommendation of the veterinarian who is able to physically evaluate your pet and knows them best.

Let us begin going through information about emergencies! I recommend you take the time to read through this book BEFORE any emergencies should strike so that you will be prepared. I will do my best to provide recommendations and suggestions for practical tools to help along the way!

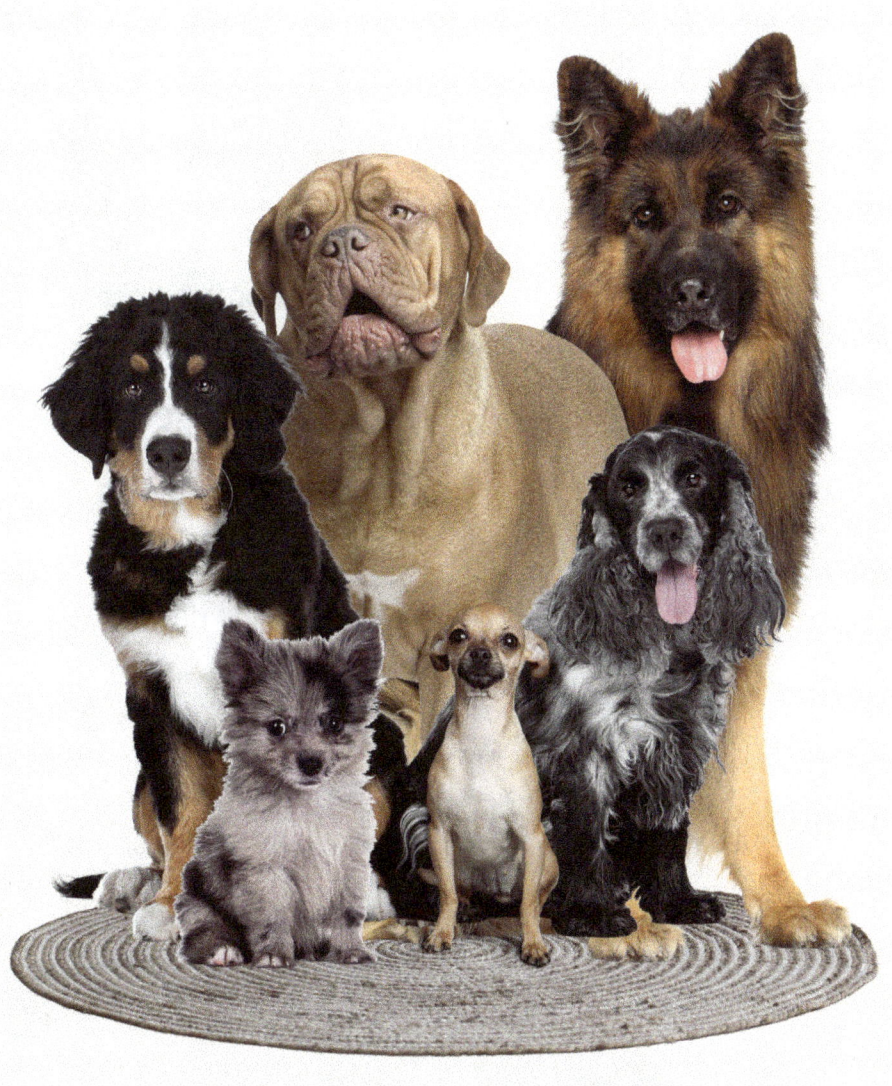

What is Your Emergency Toolkit?

Veterinary professionals use a range of techniques to assess a pet's condition and determine stability. While it takes years of training to fully master these techniques, there are key observations that pet owners can learn to help assess their pet's well-being during emergencies. Understanding and recognizing these signs will help you feel more confident in assessing whether you're facing a true emergency.

Furthermore, by observing specific indicators, you can provide your veterinarian with critical information, enabling them to offer more accurate and efficient care.

Remember, if you're ever uncertain, it's always wise to seek professional advice from a veterinarian.

Below, you'll find a quick-reference list of the key indicators in your toolkit and where to find them in the book.

TOOL	SECTION	PAGE #
Resting Respiratory Rate	Difficulty Breathing	101
Gum Moisture Assessment	Severe Vomiting/Diarrhea	107 & 149
Eye Assessment for Hydration	Severe Vomiting/Diarrhea	107 & 149
Skin Tenting	Severe Vomiting/Diarrhea	109 & 149
Capillary Refill Time	Severe Vomiting/Diarrhea	108 & 149
Pain Scale	Pain/ Difficulty Moving	137

In addition to the observations in the toolkit, which help you assess your pet's stability, I have also included guidance on how to respond when certain situations arise.

Below is a chart of the recommended responses, along with the pages where you may find more detailed information in the book.

RESPONSES	SECTION	PAGE #
Seizures	Seizures	28 & 124
Simple External Bleeding	Bleeding	120
Pain	Pain/Difficulty Moving + IVDD	134 & 114
Collapse	Collapse	131
Trauma	Trauma	123
Overheating	Heatstroke	22
Allergic Reaction	Allergic Reaction	37
Breathing Concerns	CHF + Difficulty Breathing	46 & 109
Ingestion of Foreign Material	Vomiting (Foreign Body)	73
Bite Wounds	Bite Wounds	58

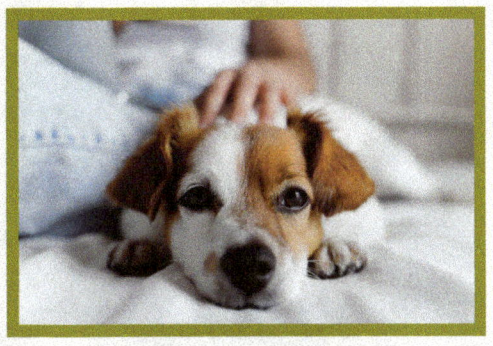

You'll find several important handouts throughout the book, designed to assist you during various stages of your pet's care. Feel free to photocopy or scan these pages for your use.

Additionally, I'm happy to provide these handouts as full-page PDFs for your convenience. You can access them on my website at www.crittercarecollective.com or simply email me at crittercarecollective@gmail.com with the subject line: "Emergency PDFs."

DOCUMENT	PURPOSE	PAGE #
First Aid Supplies Checklist	Emergency Preparation	2
Know Your Local ER Options	Emergency Preparation	4
Medical Decision Authorization Form	Emergency Preparation/ Provide to caretaker if you are away from your dog	7
Sick Visit Information Sheet	Emergency Response/ Prepare for a sick visit, to assist your veterinarian and ensure nothing is missed	9

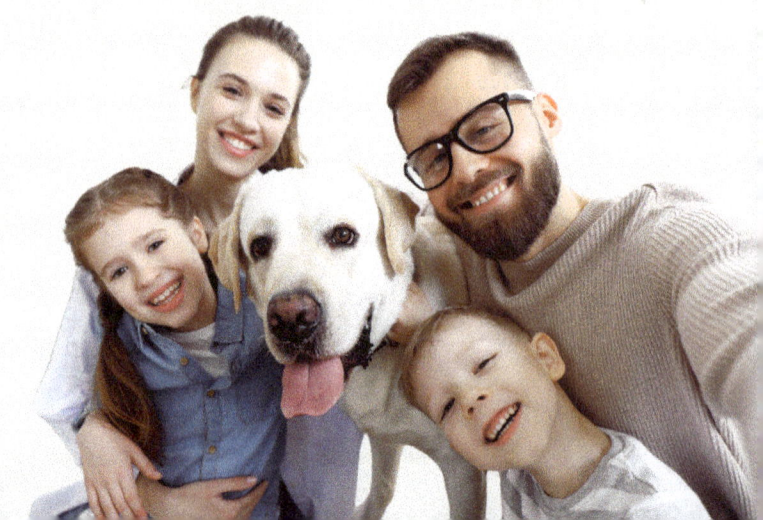

CHAPTERS

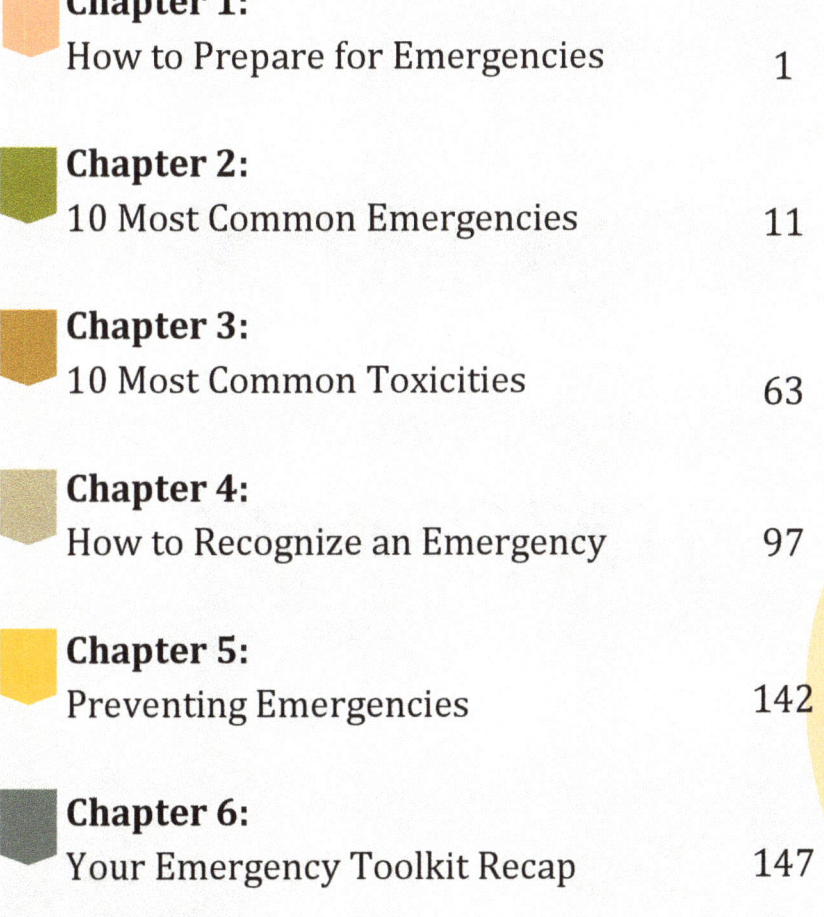

Chapter 1:
How to Prepare for Emergencies — 1

Chapter 2:
10 Most Common Emergencies — 11

Chapter 3:
10 Most Common Toxicities — 63

Chapter 4:
How to Recognize an Emergency — 97

Chapter 5:
Preventing Emergencies — 142

Chapter 6:
Your Emergency Toolkit Recap — 147

Chapter 1

HOW TO PREPARE FOR EMERGENCIES

Emergencies can happen without warning and being prepared can make all the difference when it comes to your dog's health and safety. Having a well-stocked pet first-aid kit, knowing the location of your nearest emergency vet clinic, and having an emergency plan in place are essential for managing stressful situations effectively.

In this chapter, I'll guide you through a way to put together a comprehensive pet emergency kit, the importance of planning ahead, and ways to make sure you're always prepared for the unexpected.

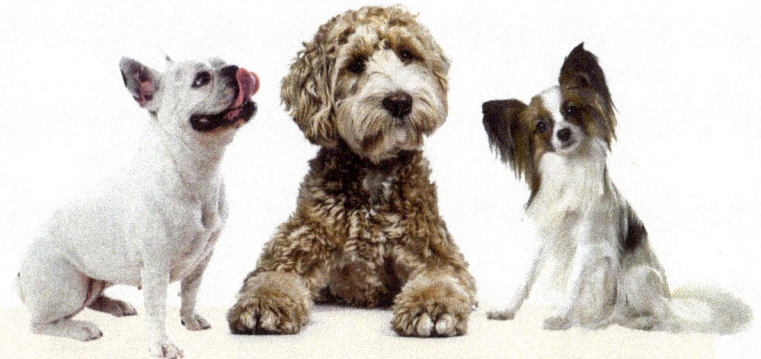

Chapter Highlights:

1. Emergency First Aid Kit Checklist

2. Knowing Your Local ER Options

3. Having an Emergency Plan

4. Preparing Your Dog for Care in Your Absence

5. Key Information for the Veterinarian

6. Pet Insurance Benefits

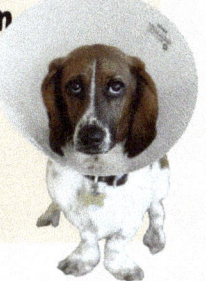

A well-equipped first-aid kit is a lifesaver in emergencies. It enables you to address common health issues and injuries right away, giving you peace of mind and the time needed to get professional help.

First Aid Supplies Checklist

Wound Care and Cleaning

Sterile Gauze Pads

Self Adhesive Bandages
i.e., Vetwrap

Wound Cleaners
 i.e., Povidone Iodine/ Betadine/ Chlorhexidine/ Saline

Cotton Balls
~Used to help clean wounds

Saline Solution

3% Hydrogen Peroxide
~In case your veterinarian recommends inducing vomiting at home

Medications and Monitoring

Medications
~ Medications prescribed for your pet

Thermometer
Rectal is best - if you are comfortable taking rectal temperatures

Cold Pack/ Hot Pack

E-Collar (Cone)
~Vital for any time we need to keep the dog from licking their body

Safety and Emergency Preparedness

First Aid Tools

Tweezers
~For removing splinters/ stingers/ticks

Disposable gloves

Safety Items

Leash and Harness

Flashlight with extra batteries
~In case you need to locate your pet in the dark

Water bowl
 - A collapsible bowl stores easily

Emergency Information

List of medications your dog takes
~Concentration, dosage, frequency

Veterinarian Contact Information
~Information for your primary veterinarian and any records you may have

Nearby Emergency Veterinary Facilities

Figure 1.1

Breakdown of Key Items in the First Aid Kit

Let's dive a little deeper into some of the items suggested for your first aid kit.

- Sterile Gauze Pads:
    - These can be applied to a wound to protect it from infection.
- Self-Adhesive Bandages (Vetwrap):
    - This stretchy bandage sticks to itself and is great for securing other dressings or providing gentle support to injuries. It can be used to secure the gauze pads in place.
    - Be aware that these should only be placed on temporarily, while you seek veterinary care. Otherwise they can cause too much pressure on the area and can make the situation worse.
- Wound Cleaners:
    - Povidone Iodine/ Betadine/ Chlorhexidine can be used to clean a wound. They will need to be <u>diluted</u> prior to use.
        - Wound cleaners may be found in most human pharmacies or purchased online.
        - Apply first to a cotton ball or gauze to clean the area.
    - NEVER use alcohol to flush a wound!
    - AVOID using hydrogen peroxide to clean the wound if it all possible. It stings and can actually delay wound healing.
    - DO NOT attempt to clean wounds that are very deep. In those cases, control bleeding and head to an emergency facility immediately.
- Hydrogen Peroxide
    - Hydrogen Peroxide should NOT be used to induce vomiting UNLESS it is under the instruction of a veterinarian/ poison control.

Know Your Local ER Options

Emergencies often occur at the worst times and your regular vet might not be available. Knowing the location and contact information of your nearest 24/7 emergency veterinary clinic is crucial to saving time and potentially saving your dog's life.

Locate Your Nearest Emergency Facility

If you are in an area with multiple ERs, locate the two that are closest to you. Ideally, ensure that at least one of the facilities you've written down is open 24/7.

Facility #1	Phone number	Address
_____	_____	_____
_____	_____	_____
Facility #2	Phone number	Address
_____	_____	_____
_____	_____	_____

Map It Out

Know the route to the Emergency Facility. If possible, drive by the location at least once to become familiar.

Save It

Save the address in your cellphone, along with your regular vet's information. You can even save the address in your GPS!

Have an Emergency Plan

Being ready for an emergency means having a plan in place in the event of an emergency. While we can't anticipate every situation, here are a few steps to consider:

- **Establish a Plan for Transporting Your Dog:**
    - If your dog is injured or in distress, have a safe method of transportation. Keep an extra leash and a towel or blanket for wrapping your dog during transport.
- **Create a List of Important Contacts:**
    - Keep with you the contact information for:
        - Your regular veterinarian
        - The nearest emergency clinic
        - ASPCA Poison Control (888-426-4435)
    - If you're traveling, it's a good idea to research emergency vet clinics along your route and keep their contact details in your car or phone.
- **Make Your Pet's Medical History Accessible:**
    - Pet records should be easily accessible. Keep a copy of your dog's medical history, vaccinations, allergies, medications, and emergency instructions in your emergency kit, on your phone, or in a digital file.
        - Ensure these get updated yearly.
    - If your dog has a pre-existing medical condition or requires special care (like daily medication), make sure that information is included. This could save time and prevent errors during an emergency.
- **Prepare for Travel with Your Pet:**
    - When you travel with your dog, always carry a portable emergency kit with travel-specific items, such as extra water, a portable bowl, leash, and any medications or your dog may need.

Preparing Your Dog for Care in Your Absence

Traveling can be stressful, especially when leaving your beloved pet in someone else's care. Sadly, emergencies can and do happen when pet owners are traveling. To ensure that your pet receives the fastest and best care while you are away, it's crucial to prepare a comprehensive document with essential information.

Key Information to Include:
1. **Basic Information**
    - Pet's name, age, and breed
    - Contact details for the owner (you)
    - Special instructions for care (diet, exercise routine, etc.)
2. **Medications and Allergies**
    - A list of all medications your pet is currently taking, including dosages and administration times
    - Any known allergies or health conditions (e.g., food allergies, sensitivities)
3. **Veterinary Contacts**
    - Name and contact information for your regular veterinarian
    - Address and phone number of a preferred emergency veterinary facility in case immediate care is needed
4. **Emergency Contact Information**
    - The best phone numbers to reach you
5. **Medical Decision-Making Authorization**
    - Specify whether the caregiver has the authority to make medical decisions on behalf of your pet in case of an emergency. <u>This can be a critical point for ensuring your pet gets the right care when needed.</u>

*A form you can use is located on the following page.

Pet Care & Medical Authorization Form

DOG'S NAME: _____

Breed: _____
Age: _____
Sex: _____

Medical Conditions, Allergies: _____
Medications (name/ dosage): _____

Dog Owner Information:
Name: _____
Address: _____
Phone number(s): _____

Caregiver Information:
Name: _____
Address: _____
Phone number(s): _____

Local Veterinarian Information:
Business Name: _____
Address: _____
Phone #: _____
Additional Information: _____

Preferred Emergency Facility:
Business Name: _____
Address: _____
Phone #: _____
Additional Information: _____

Medical Decision Making Authorization:

☐ I authorize _____[Caregiver's Name] to make medical decisions for my pet in case of an emergency if I cannot be reached.

☐ I do not authorize _____[Caregiver's Name] to make medical decisions for my pet in case of an emergency if I cannot be reached.

Completed by: _____ Date: _____

Figure 1.2

Prepare Key Information to Share with the Vet

When you contact the vet or emergency clinic, they'll need specific information to assess the situation and guide their next steps. If you come prepared with this information, this can be very helpful. Some things to have in mind:

Your Pet's Identification Information:

- Your dog's name, age, breed
- Any pre-existing medical conditions, current medications, or allergies that might be relevant.

Symptoms and Timeline:

- Describe your dog's symptoms as clearly and specifically as possible (e.g., "Vomiting once every two hours," or "Limping after jumping off the couch").
- Let them know when the symptoms started or when the incident (like an injury or exposure to toxins) occurred.
- Do the best you can to provide the information in a logical timeline, as if you were telling a story.

Any Treatments Tried:

- Inform the vet of anything you've already attempted.

Potential Causes or Exposures:

- Provide any relevant information you know.
    - For example: your dog ingested something; there was known trauma; there was exposure to sick animals; etc.

Behavioral Changes or Concerns:

- Remember, dogs may act differently at the veterinary facility. It is important for us to know of any unusual behaviors you are observing.
- Also, no one knows your dog like you do! If something seems concerning/abnormal to you, we want to know!

Figure 1.3: Information to gather for your veterinarian when your dog is sick

SICK VISIT INFO

DOG'S NAME: _____

BREED: _____ AGE: _____ MALE/ FEMALE   INTACT/ ALTERED

EXISTING MEDICAL CONDITIONS:

CURRENT MEDICATIONS:

SYMPTOMS:
Include when signs started

ANY KNOWN/ SUSPECTED CAUSES:

TREATMENTS ALREADY ATTEMPTED:

OTHER CONCERNS:

Printable versions of this chart are available at crittercarecollective.com

Pet Insurance Benefits

As a devoted dog owner, you want the best for your dog. But unexpected veterinary costs can add up quickly, especially during emergencies. Pet insurance can be a valuable financial safety net, providing peace of mind and helping to manage veterinary expenses.

- Financial Protection Against High Costs
    - Emergency care for dogs can be incredibly expensive. Pet insurance can cover a significant portion of these costs, making care more accessible.
- Access to Quality Care
    - With pet insurance, you can make decisions based on your dog's health needs rather than your financial situation. This can lead to better outcomes, as you won't have to hesitate to seek necessary treatments.
- Preventive Care Options
    - Many pet insurance plans offer coverage for preventive care, such as vaccinations, routine check-ups, and dental cleanings, which can help keep your dog healthy and avoid costly illnesses down the line.

Enroll When Your Dog is Young and Healthy

The best time to get pet insurance is when your dog is young. Premiums are generally lower, and coverage is more comprehensive since your dog won't have preexisting conditions that could lead to exclusions.

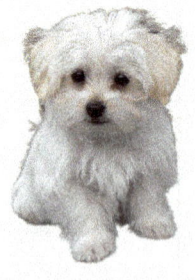

It's important to note that most pet insurance policies do not cover preexisting conditions. If your dog is diagnosed with an illness before enrollment, any related treatment will likely be excluded from coverage.

Many veterinary pet insurance companies exist. Be sure to talk to your veterinarian about your needs and recommended pet insurance option.

Chapter 2

TEN MOST COMMON EMERGENCIES

Emergencies can happen without warning and knowing how to handle them is crucial for any pet owner. In this chapter, we'll focus on the top ten emergencies every dog owner should be prepared to face - from common issues like back pain to more serious situations like bloat (GDV). You'll learn how to recognize the signs, understand the causes, and take the right steps in those critical moments.

Chapter Highlights

Top 10 Emergencies:

1. Spinal Pain
2. Trauma
3. Heatstroke
4. Seizures
5. Bloat
6. Allergic Reactions
7. Hemoabdomen (Abdominal bleeding)
8. Congestive Heart Failure
9. Vomiting-- Foreign Body
10. Bite Wounds

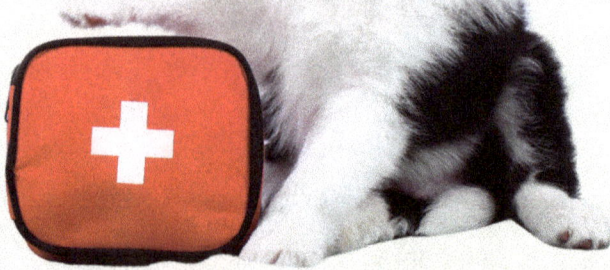

Emergency #1

SPINAL PAIN

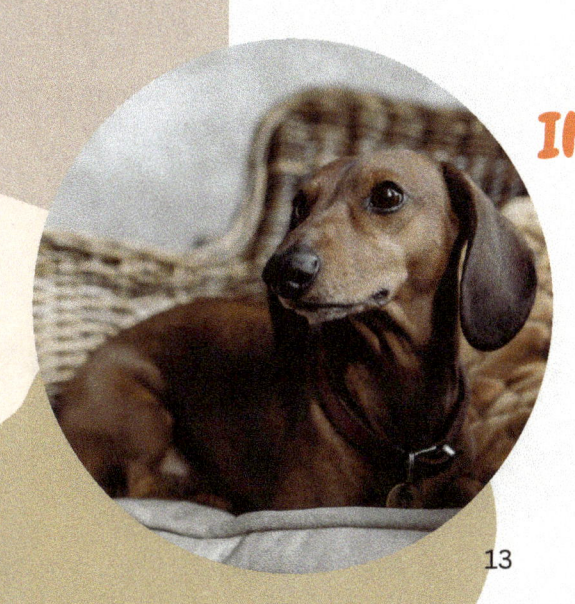

INTERVERTEBRAL DISC DISEASE (IVDD)

What is Intervertebral Disc Disease (IVDD)?

Intervertebral Disc Disease (IVDD) affects the discs between the vertebrae in a dog's spine. When these discs degenerate (wear down) or herniate (disc material pushes out - similar to "slipped disc" in humans), they can press on the spinal cord, causing pain, weakness, or paralysis. Not all spinal pain is due to IVDD, but since it is a fairly common cause of signs, we will discuss it here.

Dogs Most Affected

Breeds predisposed to Intervertebral Disc Disease (IVDD) include:

1. Dachshunds
2. Beagles
3. Corgis
4. Basset Hounds
5. Shih Tzus
6. French Bulldogs
7. Pekingese
8. Bulldogs (English and American)

While these breeds are at higher risk, IVDD can occur in any dog.

Dogs are predisposed due to genetics, age (with older dogs having a higher risk), obesity, exposure to repetitive motion stress, and injury.

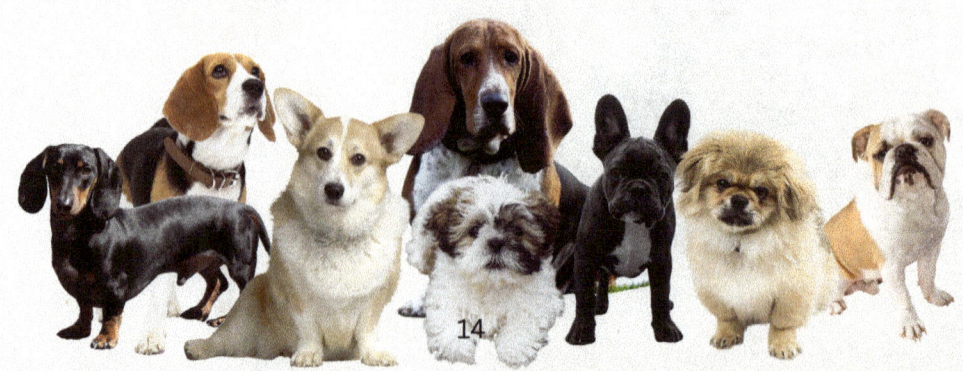

Signs of IVDD

IVDD signs vary based on severity. Some common signs include:

- **Back Pain:** Reluctance to move, yelping when touched, or an arched back.
- **Hunched Posture:** Dogs may adopt a hunched stance to minimize pain.
- **Difficulty with Stairs/Jumping**: People often report avoidance of stairs and reluctance to jump.
- **Difficulty Walking:** Unsteady gait or weakness in the hind legs.
  - If severe, the hind legs may become paralyzed.
- **Muscle Spasms**: Visible twitching or spasms in the back.
- **Loss of Bladder Control:** Severe cases may lead to incontinence.
  - In these situations, the dogs are usually also paralyzed in the hind legs.

What Can You Do?

If you suspect back pain, please do the following:
1. Limit Activity: Keep your dog calm and prevent jumping or running. If they are crate trained, place them in the crate.
    a. Limit walks to using the bathroom only. No long walks.
2. Contact Your Veterinarian Immediately: Describe the observed signs to assess urgency.
3. Avoid Manipulating the Spine: Do not stretch or manipulate your dog's back.

Common Interventions:

At the veterinary clinic/hospital, you may expect the following:
- Veterinary Examination: This includes a thorough exam and discussion of history.
  - For a complete diagnosis, an MRI may be needed, which will typically require a neurologist.
- Medications: Pain relief and anti-inflammatory medications will manage discomfort.
- Rest: Strict crate rest may be recommended for healing.
- Surgery: In severe cases, surgery may be necessary to relieve spinal cord pressure.
- Physical Therapy: Rehabilitation exercises will promote strength and mobility once pain is managed.

Prevention

IVDD may not always be preventable. However, some things that may help include:

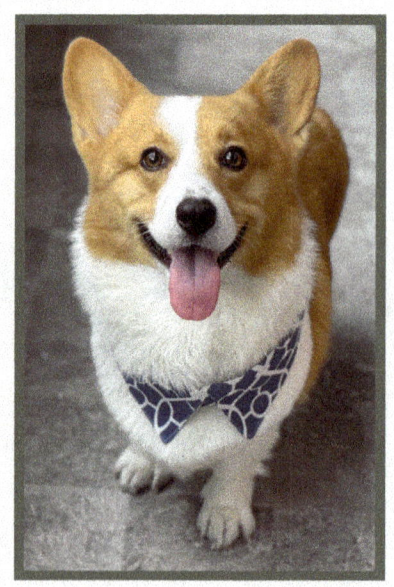

- Maintaining a Healthy Weight: This helps alleviate stress on the spine and is especially important for breeds at high risk.
- Limit High-Risk Activities: Avoid excessive jumping or rough play with prone breeds.
- Provide Proper Support: Use ramps to minimize jumping into cars or onto furniture.

Emergency #2

TRAUMA

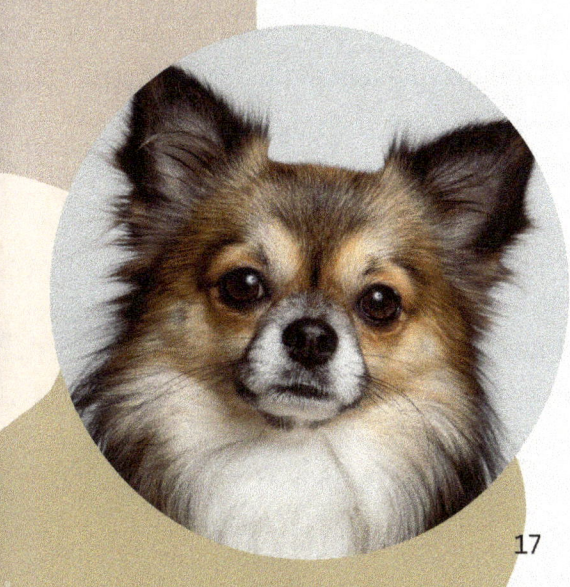

What is Trauma?

Trauma in dogs refers to injuries that occur due to accidents, fights, falls, or vehicle collisions. These injuries can range from minor cuts to serious conditions requiring immediate veterinary attention. Please reference the previous chapter to consider some signs that indicate that trauma may be a more immediate emergency. Reference Chapter Four for more indicators of trauma severity.

Dogs Most Affected

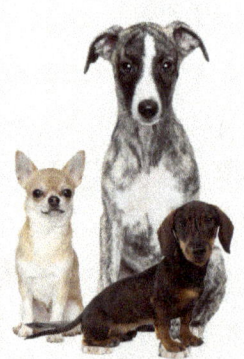

Trauma can happen to any dog. However, some breeds and individual dogs may be more affected by trauma. Small dogs (such as Chihuahuas or Dachshunds) or dogs with thin, long legs (such as Italian Greyhounds or Whippets) are more sensitive to trauma when it occurs.

Dogs with very high energy are more likely to run out of the house or escape their leash and are more prone to vehicular trauma.

Signs of Trauma

Being aware of the signs of trauma can help you act quickly. They include:

- Limping or Inability to Move: If your dog is limping, has trouble walking, or suddenly can't move, this is a red flag.
- Bleeding: Look for bleeding from the mouth, nose, or any wounds on their body.
- Swelling or Bruising: Swollen areas or bruising can indicate internal injuries or soft tissue damage.
- Unconsciousness or Confusion: If your dog is unresponsive or seems disoriented, it's a serious situation.
- Signs of Pain: Whining, yelping, hiding, or adopting unusual postures can all indicate that your dog is in pain.

What Can You Do?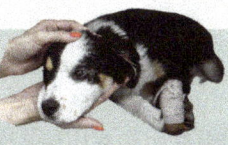

If your dog experiences *minor* trauma only and appears to be otherwise comfortable and stable, follow these steps:
1. <u>Minimize Activity:</u> Put your dog in a crate or small room to limit movement. No running, jumping, or stairs should be allowed.
2. <u>Contact your Veterinarian:</u> Provide your veterinarian with information about the trauma and the signs you are seeing. Follow their guidance for care.

If your dog experiences *major* trauma, follow these steps:
1. <u>Keep Your Pet Still:</u> Minimize handling your dog, especially if there is concern for spinal trauma. Moving your dog may worsen the injury. Keep them as still as possible until transporting.
2. <u>Control Bleeding:</u> If bleeding is present, apply direct pressure to the wound using a clean cloth or gauze to help stop it.
3. <u>Check Responsiveness:</u> If, following trauma, your dog seems to be confused/dazed/poorly responsive, this is an emergency and veterinary care is needed without delay.

<u>Transport Safely:</u> Get your dog to the veterinarian as quickly and safely as possible. If there's a chance that the neck or back was hurt during the injury, support those structures while transporting.

Regardless of the type of trauma or intervention selected, it is important to monitor your dog closely for the next few days following trauma. Some signs, like breathing difficulties, may have a delayed onset. This means that signs may develop a few days after the trauma itself.

Common Interventions:

While each case is different, here are some common interventions relative to trauma that are to be expected at the veterinary hospital, depending on each dog's needs:

1. Physical Examination: a thorough assessment to check for visible injuries, pain response, and overall health status
2. Diagnostic Imaging: X-rays or ultrasounds to evaluate for fractures, internal injuries, or foreign bodies
3. Wound Care: cleaning, suturing, or bandaging wounds to prevent infection and promote healing
4. Pain Management: administering analgesics or anti-inflammatory medications to manage pain and discomfort
5. Stabilization: providing fluids, oxygen, or other supportive care for shock or severe injuries
6. Splinting: applying a splint for fractures as needed to immobilize the affected area
7. Surgery: wound closure using surgical sutures or staples
8. Blood Tests: conducting blood work to assess organ function, blood loss, or infection
9. Neurological Assessment: evaluating neurological function if there are signs of head trauma or spinal injury
10. Monitoring: keeping the pet under observation for vital signs, response to treatment, and recovery progress

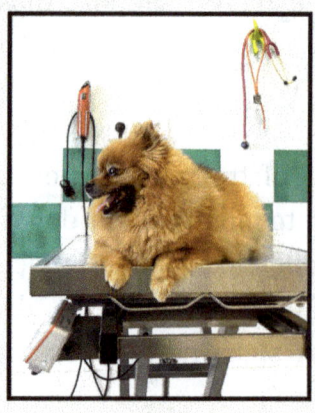

Prevention

While some trauma is unavoidable, consider the following strategies:

- Leash Training: Always keep your dog on a leash in public areas to prevent them from running into traffic or hazardous situations. Use a well-fitted collar or harness.
- Secure Fencing: Ensure your yard is securely fenced to prevent your dog from escaping and wandering into danger, such as busy roads.
- Supervised Outdoor Time: When outside, supervise your dog closely to prevent accidents, especially in unfenced areas or during play.
- Safe Walking Practices: Be vigilant while walking your dog near roads. Choose routes with sidewalks and cross streets at designated crosswalks.
- Use Reflective Gear: Equip your dog with a reflective collar or harness, especially for walks in low-light conditions, to increase visibility to drivers.
- Training Commands: Teach important commands like "come" and "stay" to help keep your dog safe in potentially dangerous situations.
- Avoid High-Risk Activities: Supervise your dog during high-energy play or activities near obstacles that could lead to falls or injuries.
- Regular Vet Check-Ups: Ensure your dog is healthy and fit for physical activity as underlying health issues can increase the risk of accidents.
- Pet-Proofing Your Home: Remove hazards around the house, such as loose cables, sharp objects, or unstable furniture, to prevent falls or injuries indoors.

Emergency #3

HEATSTROKE

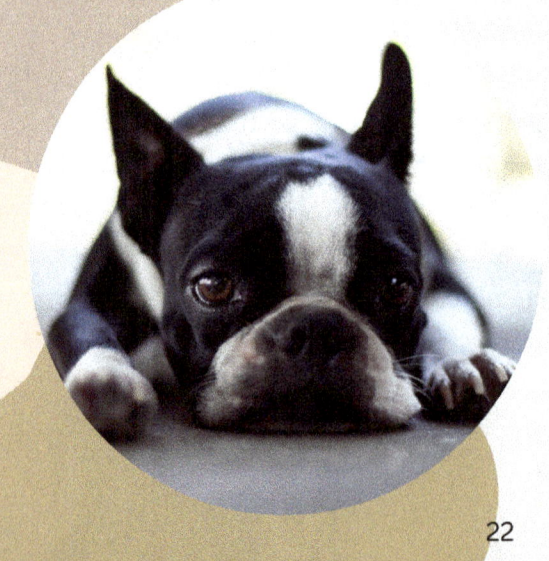

What is Heatstroke?

Heatstroke occurs when a dog's body temperature rises to dangerous levels and they can't cool down effectively. This condition can escalate quickly, leading to breakdown of body proteins and possibility of organ damage. This condition is highly dangerous and can be fatal.

Dogs Most Affected

Heatstroke can happen to <u>any</u> dog that is exposed to overly hot temperatures for a prolonged time period. Most common scenarios include dogs who have gone on long walks on hot days and dogs left in cars on hot days.

Some dogs are at a higher risk. Those include:

- <u>Brachycephalic Breeds:</u> Dogs with short noses, such as Bulldogs, Pugs, and Shih Tzus, have difficulty breathing and regulating temperature.

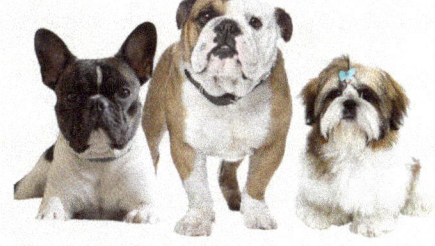

- <u>Obese Dogs:</u> Extra weight can hinder a dog's ability to cool down.

- <u>Elderly or Very Young Dogs:</u> Puppies and senior dogs may struggle with temperature regulation.

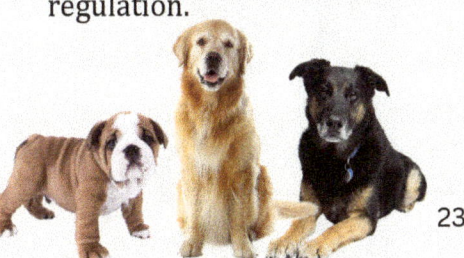

- <u>Dogs with Certain Health Conditions:</u> Those with heart or respiratory issues are at greater risk.

Signs of Heatstroke

Recognizing the signs early is crucial. Look out for:
- **Excessive Panting and Drooling:** Your dog may pant heavily and drool more than usual as they attempt to regulate their body temperature.
- **Weakness or Collapse:** If your dog seems lethargic or suddenly collapses, it's a serious concern.
  - **Bright Red or Pale Gums:** Check your dog's gums - they should be a healthy pink. Bright red or pale gums indicate distress (See Fig 2.1 for an example of pale gums).
- **Vomiting or Diarrhea:** Gastrointestinal upset can occur as a response to heat stress.
- **Rapid Heartbeat or Breathing:** An increased heart rate or difficulty breathing are alarming signs.
- **Seizures or Disorientation**: Confusion and disorientation may happen due to electrolyte imbalances and damage to brain function due to heat.

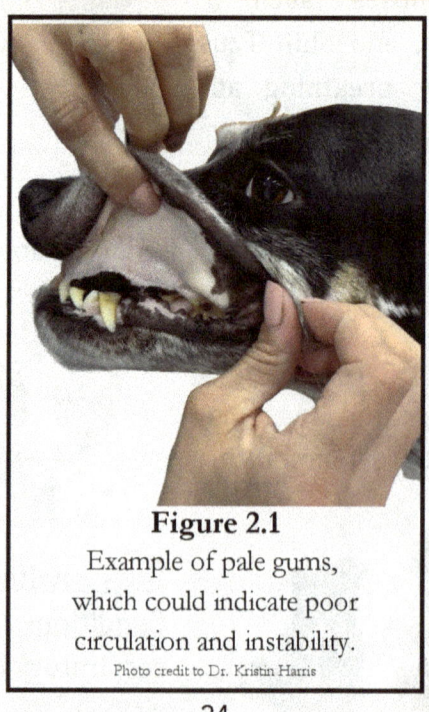

Figure 2.1
Example of pale gums, which could indicate poor circulation and instability.
Photo credit to Dr. Kristin Harris

What Can You Do?

If you suspect your dog is experiencing heatstroke, act quickly!
1. **Move your dog to a cool, shaded area** to prevent further temperature increase.
2. **Offer cool water** (but not ice-cold). Offer small sips.
    a. DO NOT attempt to force water into the mouth.
3. **Wet your dog's body and neck** with cool water or wrap them in a cool, damp towel.
    a. Note: Using <u>ice water</u> can cause the blood vessels near the skin to constrict (narrow), hence leading to trapping heat inside the body, rather than cooling. Always use cool water, but not ice-cold water.
4. **Use a fan** to enhance evaporative cooling. Avoid using ice or very cold water, as this can lead to shock.
5. **Transport to an emergency veterinarian** regardless of their immediate improvement!

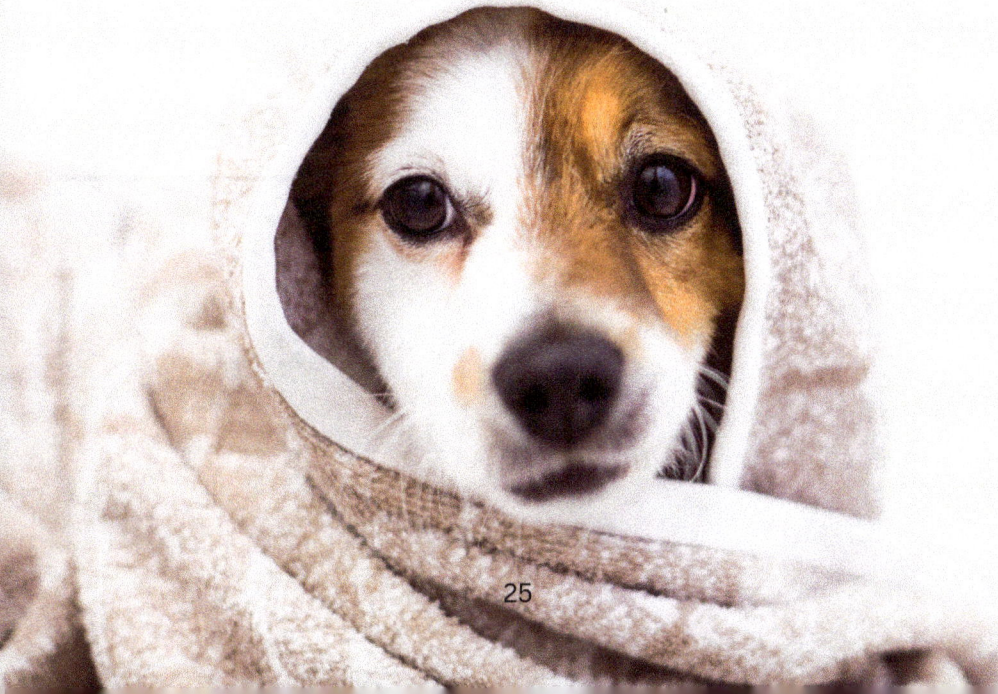

Common Interventions:

While each case is different, here are some common interventions relative to heatstroke that are to be expected at the veterinary hospital:

- <u>Immediate Assessment:</u> The vet will quickly check the dog's vital signs, including temperature, heart rate, and breathing.
- <u>Cooling Measures:</u> The dog is cooled down using methods like applying cool (not cold) water, fans, or ice packs to key areas (like the neck, armpits, and groin).
  - Cooling is done in a very precise manner to ensure the temperature is not dropped too low or too quickly!
- <u>Oxygen Therapy:</u> Oxygen support is often provided during this process to support breathing.
- <u>Intravenous (IV) Fluids:</u> IV fluids are often given to further help cooling as well as to rehydrate the dog and restore electrolyte balance.
- <u>Bloodwork:</u> Blood parameters are often checked to ensure that proteins have not broken down and that the ability to clot is not diminished.
- <u>Monitoring:</u> Continuous monitoring of vital signs and neurological status is performed to assess recovery and detect any complications.
- <u>Additional Treatments:</u> Depending on the severity, further treatments may include medications to manage symptoms, prevent shock, or address organ damage. A plasma transfusion may be needed if clotting deficiencies are found.

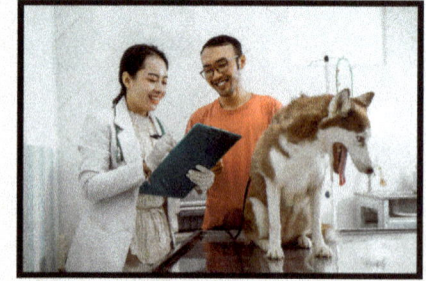

Prevention

Preventing heatstroke is essential for your dog's health. Here are some key tips:

- **Never leave your dog in a hot car.** Even with the windows cracked, the temperature inside a car can rise dangerously high within minutes.

- **Avoid exercise during peak heat.** Plan walks and playtime during cooler parts of the day, like early morning or late evening.

- **Provide access to an indoor area.** Dogs left outside on hot days may overheat rapidly, even if they are not exercising.

- **Provide fresh water and shade.** Ensure your dog has access to plenty of fresh water and shade during outdoor activities to keep them cool.

A study conducted by the Stanford University Medical Center found that the temperature within a car may increase to an average of 40° above the outside temperature within just one hour, with the majority of the heat increasing in the first 15 to 30 minutes. (See Fig 2.2 for a representation of expected car temperatures on hot days.)

Note that cracking windows open did not significantly reduce the car temperature.

Outside Temp (°F)	Car Temp (°F)
70°F	110°F
80°F	120°F
90°F	130°F

Figure 2.2: Table providing visual representation of approximate increases in car temperature within 1 hour

Heatstroke is a preventable condition, but it can escalate quickly. By recognizing the signs and taking immediate action, you can protect your dog's health and ensure they stay safe during hot weather.

Emergency #4

SEIZURES

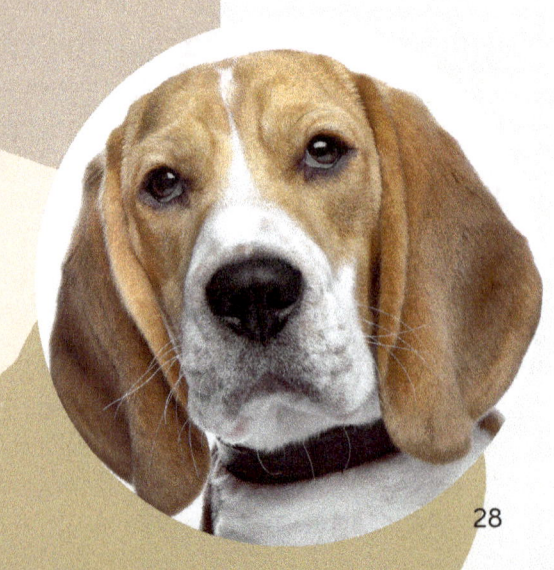

What Are Seizures?

Seizures in dogs are sudden, uncontrolled electrical disturbances in the brain, often caused by neurological issues, exposure to toxins, or underlying medical conditions. Recognizing the signs and knowing how to respond is vital for your dog's safety.

Dogs Most Affected

Any dog can develop seizures. But some dogs are more prone to them due to genetic factors, neurological conditions, and underlying health issues. Some dog breeds with seemingly higher seizure risk include:

1. Beagle
2. German Shepherd
3. Labrador Retriever
4. Siberian Husky
5. Boxer
6. Cocker Spaniel
7. Border Collie
8. Dalmatian
9. Poodle
10. Australian Shepherd

In addition to breed, other factors such as age (with younger dogs often experiencing idiopathic epilepsy), certain medical conditions, and exposure to toxins can also contribute to seizure likelihood.

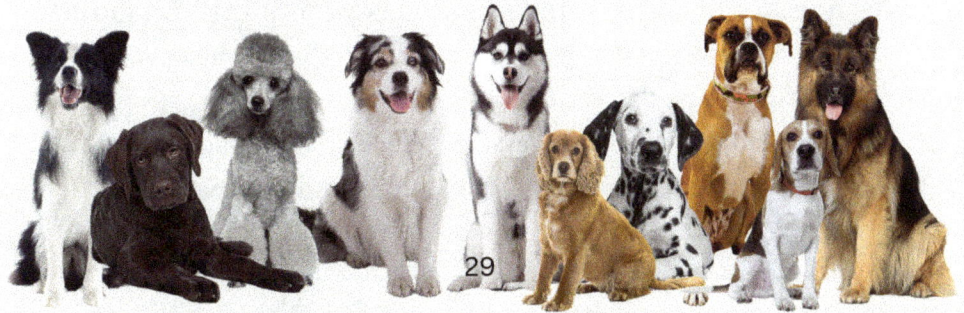

Signs of Seizures

Refer back to the first chapter discussing the types of seizures and phases. As a recap, some signs a seizure may have occurred include:

- **Sudden Collapse**: Your dog may suddenly fall over or lose balance.
- **Jerking or Twitching:** Look for uncontrollable movements, twitching, or stiffening of the body.
- **Stiffening of Neck/ Limbs:** Oftentimes the legs or neck will become rigid and extend during the event.
- **Loss of Consciousness:** During a seizure, your dog may be unresponsive and unaware of their surroundings.
- **Foaming at the Mouth**: Excessive drooling or foaming can occur, along with loss of bladder control.
- **Post-Seizure Confusion (Postictal State):** After a seizure, your dog might seem disoriented, confused, or excessively tired.

What Can You Do?

If your dog is having a seizure, here's what you can do:
1. **Keep Your Dog Safe:** Move any sharp objects or hazards away from your dog to prevent injury during the seizure.
2. **Do Not Put Anything in Their Mouth:** Contrary to popular belief, do not try to hold their tongue or put anything in their mouth as this can cause injury to both you and your dog.
3. **Time the Seizure:** If the seizure lasts more than 5 minutes, seek emergency veterinary care immediately, as prolonged seizures can be dangerous.
4. **Calm and Rest:** After the seizure, help your dog calm down and allow them to rest in a quiet, comfortable place.

(See Fig. 6.8 at the end of the book for further guidance.)

Common Interventions:

Some expected interventions for seizures administered by the vet include:
1. <u>Physical Examination:</u> a thorough assessment to check for any signs of trauma, neurological deficits, or other health issues
2. <u>History Taking</u>: documenting precise history about the seizure episodes, including frequency, duration, and any triggers or accompanying symptoms
3. <u>Blood Tests</u>: checking metabolic issues, infections, or organ dysfunction that could contribute to seizures
4. <u>Neurological Assessment:</u> evaluating the pet's neurological status, including reflexes, coordination, and responsiveness
5. <u>Diagnostic Imaging:</u> performing X-rays/ultrasound to assess for extracranial (outside of the brain) causes for the seizure
6. <u>Immediate Seizure Management</u>: Administering medications, such as benzodiazepines (e.g., diazepam or midazolam) to control active seizures and prevent further episodes
7. <u>Long-term Medication</u>: discussing options for anticonvulsant medications if seizures are frequent or severe, including phenobarbital, levetiracetam, or others
8. <u>Monitoring:</u> keeping the pet under observation to assess response to treatment and monitor for any side effects
9. <u>Referral to Specialists:</u> Evaluation by a neurologist may be recommended. This will include an MRI to assess for intracranial (inside the brain) causes for the seizures.

Prevention

There is no way to prevent seizures from happening. But being aware of the possibility of seizures and responding, as needed, is critical. Additionally, if your pet has seizures and is on medications, <u>do not</u> discontinue them without veterinarian recommendation.

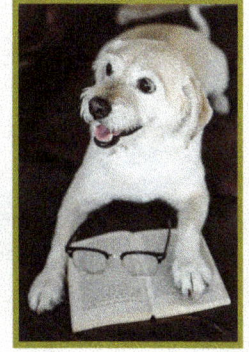

Emergency #5

BLOAT
(GDV)

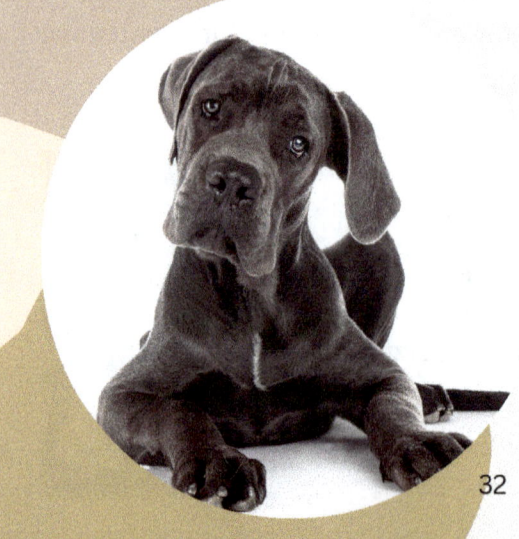

What is Bloat?

Bloat, or Gastric Dilatation-Volvulus (GDV), is a serious and potentially life-threatening condition that commonly occurs in large, deep-chested dogs. It happens when the stomach fills with gas, food, or fluid, and then twists on itself, trapping the contents and cutting off blood flow to the stomach and nearby organs. This condition is a surgical emergency and prompt care is essential.

Dogs Most Affected

Certain breeds are more predisposed to developing bloat. These include:
1. Great Dane
2. German Shepherd
3. Boxer
4. Rottweiler
5. Doberman Pinscher
6. Weimaraner
7. Siberian Husky
8. Standard Poodle
9. Irish Setter
10. Basset Hound

While these breeds are at higher risk, bloat can occur in <u>any dog</u>. Factors such as age, diet, and family history also play a role.

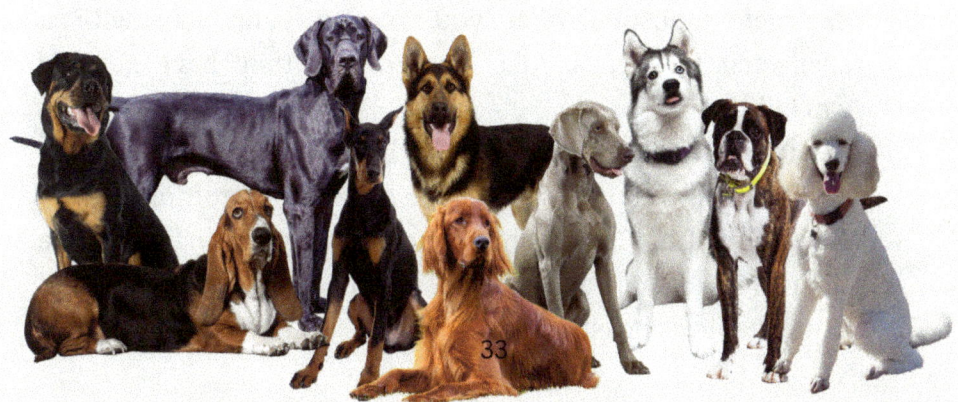

Signs of GDV

GDV leads to a combination of signs due to the rapidly distending abdomen and twisted stomach.

- **Distended/Swollen Abdomen:** The belly appears visibly bloated or distended, often firm to the touch.
- **Unsuccessful Vomiting:** Your dog may retch or try to vomit while unable to bring up anything.
- **Restlessness:** Dogs with bloat may pace, seem anxious, or have difficulty finding a comfortable position.
- **Rapid Breathing:** An increased respiratory rate is commonly seen due to distress.
- **Drooling:** Excessive saliva production may occur as the dog struggles with discomfort.
- **Weakness or Lethargy:** A sudden drop in energy levels can be a significant warning sign.

These signs are rapidly progressive and will quickly lead to complications such as shock, cardiac arrest, and death if not addressed immediately.

What Can You Do?

If you suspect your dog has a GDV, act quickly:
1. **Seek Emergency Veterinary Care**: Call ahead to inform the emergency hospital that you are on your way with a suspected GDV case. Also, ensure that they have surgery capabilities.
2. **Avoid Feeding or Giving Water:** Do not try to feed your dog or give them water, as this could worsen the condition.
3. **Keep Your Dog Calm:** While transporting your dog, minimize their movement and stress. Keep them as still and comfortable as possible.

Common Interventions:

Once at the veterinary clinic, the following treatments may occur relative to GDV:

- Stabilization: Your dog will likely receive intravenous fluids to stabilize their condition.
- X-Rays: The veterinarian may perform an X-Ray to confirm the GDV and assess the extent of the situation (See Fig 2.3).
- Decompression: The vet may relieve some pressure in the stomach by passing a large needle or catheter into the stomach, through the side of the body, or through passing a tube into the stomach through the mouth.
- Surgery: Surgical intervention is required to untwist the stomach and tack the stomach in place to prevent it from twisting again.
    - Depending on the degree of tissue damage in the area, pieces of the stomach and the spleen may also need to be removed.

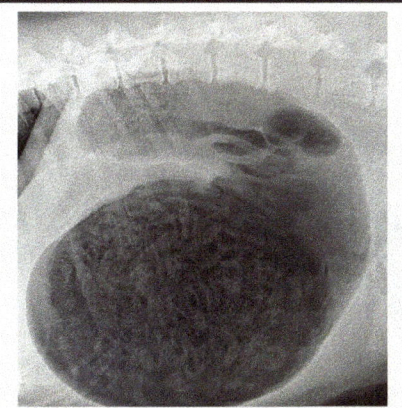

X-ray showing a "double bubble" appearance, classic for a GDV.

This image is of Walter, a 5-year-old castrated male Bernese Mountain Dog who belongs to a family of veterinarians. Even vets have emergencies and Walter had to visit an Emergency Veterinarian. Thankfully, Walter made a full recovery!

Photo credit to Mt Washington Animal Clinic

Figure 2.3

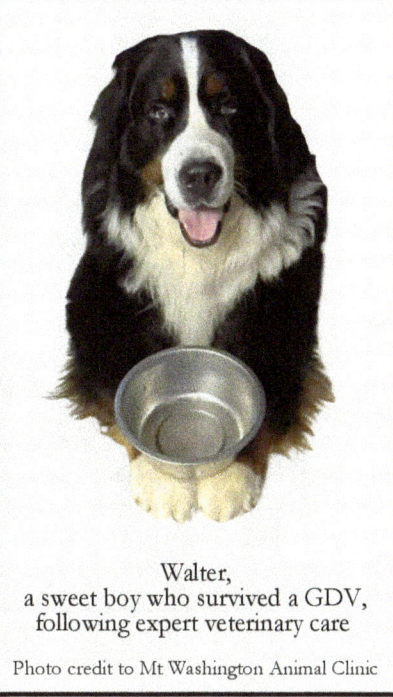

Walter,
a sweet boy who survived a GDV, following expert veterinary care

Photo credit to Mt Washington Animal Clinic

Prevention

There is ongoing research being conducted to try to understand exactly WHY a GDV occurs, and hence, how to prevent it. However, some recommendations exist and are listed below:

- **Consider Gastropexy**: If your dog is at high risk for GDV, talk to your veterinarian about a preventive gastropexy. This surgical procedure attaches the stomach to the abdominal wall, making it less likely to twist.
- **Avoid** feeding from an elevated bowl (increases air swallowing).
- **Avoid** feeding large amounts of food at one time.
- **Consider Methods to Slow Down Eating:** With a goal to decrease the amount of air swallowed during feeding, eating more slowly/calmly and eating a smaller amount (more frequently) is ideal.

Ultimately, a GDV is not truly preventable. Being aware of the signs involved and responding quickly is crucial.

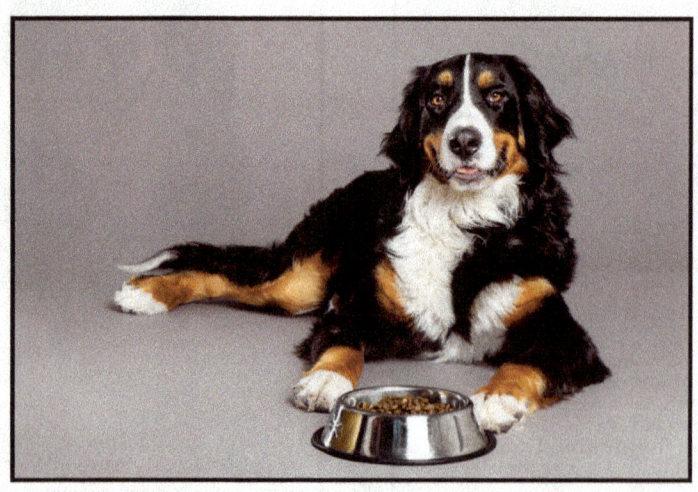

Emergency #6

ALLERGIC REACTIONS

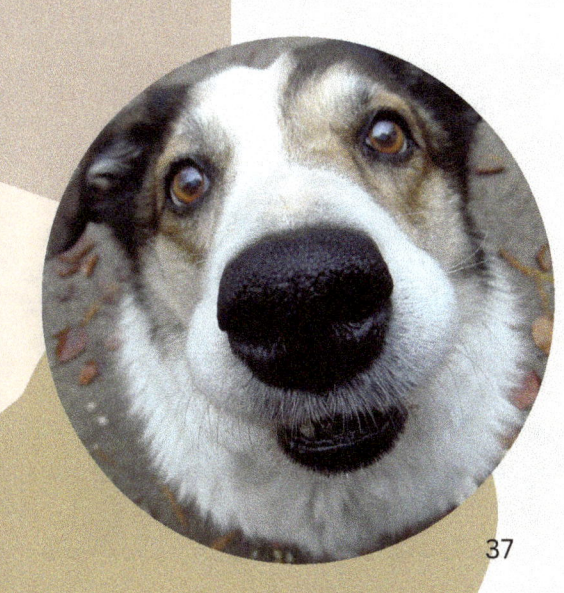

What are Allergic Reactions (Acute Hypersensitivity Reactions)?

Dogs can experience allergic reactions to various triggers, including certain foods, medications, vaccines, and environmental factors like insect stings. The dog's immune system overreacts and releases inflammatory substances, which lead to the reaction.

Fortunately, most allergic reactions seen in the emergency room tend to be fairly mild.

Dogs Most Affected

Certain dog breeds are more predisposed to acute hypersensitivity reactions, including those triggered by vaccines, medications, or environmental allergens. Those are:

1. Boxers
2. Bulldogs (English and French)
3. Retrievers (Golden and Labrador)
4. Cocker Spaniels
5. Schnauzers
6. Dachshunds
7. Shetland Sheepdogs
8. Beagles
9. Poodles (all sizes)
10. Yorkshire Terriers

Any dog can develop an allergic reaction.

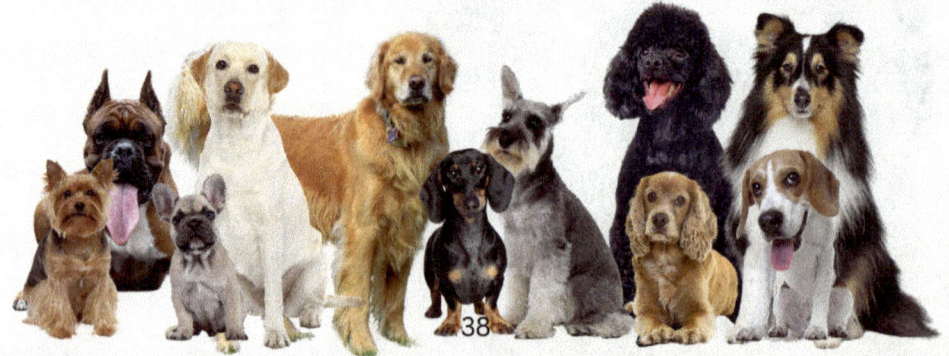

Signs of Allergic Reactions

Be on the lookout for these signs:
- **Swelling**: Look for swelling in the face, lips, or around the eyes.
- **Hives or Itchy Skin:** Red, itchy patches or hives can appear on your dog's skin (See Fig 2.4).
  - Often these will be seen around the belly/hind legs/top of head, but they can be anywhere.
- **Difficulty Breathing:** Any signs of labored or noisy breathing should be taken seriously. Thankfully this is not common.
- **Gastrointestinal Issues**: Symptoms like vomiting, diarrhea, or excessive drooling may occur and may indicate more profound disease.
- **Lethargy or Collapse:** If your dog seems unusually tired or collapses, it's a critical sign of distress.

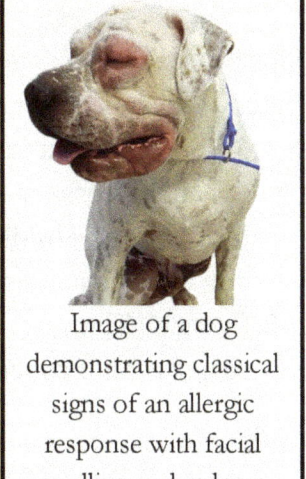

Image of a dog demonstrating classical signs of an allergic response with facial swelling and redness

Photo credit to Animal Emergency Hospital, Burton, MI

Figure 2.4

What Can You Do?

1. Contact Your Veterinarian: Severe allergic reactions can lead to anaphylaxis, a life-threatening condition that requires urgent care.
2. Administer Antihistamines (if advised): Only give antihistamines that your vet has recommended for emergencies. Do not administer over-the-counter medications without guidance.
3. Monitor Breathing: If you suspect labored breathing, get your pet to a veterinary clinic immediately.
4. Seek Veterinary Care: If signs are profound or there is suspicion for anaphylaxis, immediately seek vet care.

Common Interventions

Some expected interventions by the vet for allergic reactions include:
1. <u>Antihistamines:</u> Medications like diphenhydramine (Benadryl) can help alleviate mild allergic symptoms. At the veterinarian, this is usually given initially as an injection.
2. <u>Corticosteroids:</u> For more severe reactions, corticosteroids can reduce inflammation and immune response.

Most cases are treated on an outpatient model. IF anaphylaxis is noted (which is not very common), interventions may include:
1. <u>Epinephrine</u>: In cases of anaphylaxis, an epinephrine injection may be necessary to rapidly counteract severe reactions.
2. <u>Intravenous Fluids:</u> Administering IV fluids can help stabilize a dog experiencing shock or severe allergic reactions.
3. <u>Oxygen Therapy</u>: Oxygen may be provided to assist with respiration if concerns are noted.

Prevention

- **Avoid Known Allergens:** If the substance that your dog reacted to is known, avoidance is key.
- **Be Prepared:** In particular, if your dog has had an allergic reaction in the past, talking to your veterinarian about antihistamines that are safe to use at home can expedite a response and resolution of signs.
- **Pre-medicate Prior to Vaccines:** If your dog has shown reactions to vaccines, your vet may opt to pre-medicate with an antihistamine prior to the next vaccine.

   Your veterinarian may also want to administer vaccines on different days and not at the same time.

Emergency #7

HEMOABDOMEN
(BLOOD IN THE ABDOMEN)

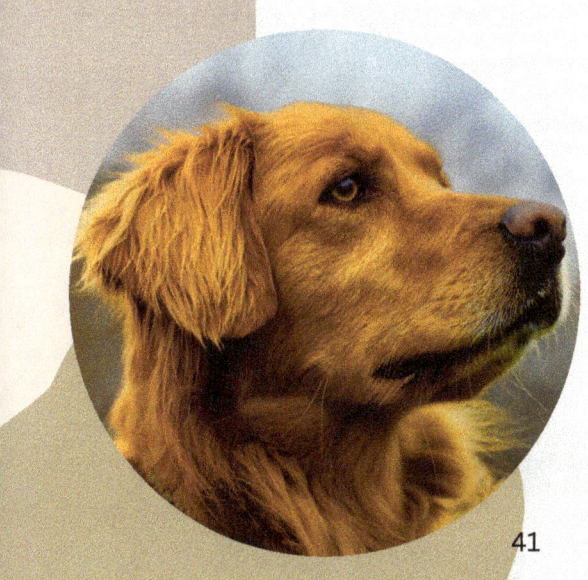

What is Hemoabdomen?

Hemoabdomen refers to the accumulation of blood in the abdominal cavity of dogs. This condition can occur due to various reasons, including tumors, trauma, or clotting disorders. Hemoabdomen is a serious medical issue that requires prompt veterinary attention.

Dogs Most Affected

Certain dog breeds are more predisposed to developing hemoabdomen. Those are:

1. Golden Retriever
2. Labrador Retriever
3. German Shepherd
4. Boxer
5. Rottweiler
6. Siberian Husky
7. Dalmatian
8. Weimaraner
9. Bernese Mountain Dog
10. Airedale Terrier

While these breeds are at higher risk, hemoabdomen can occur in any dog.

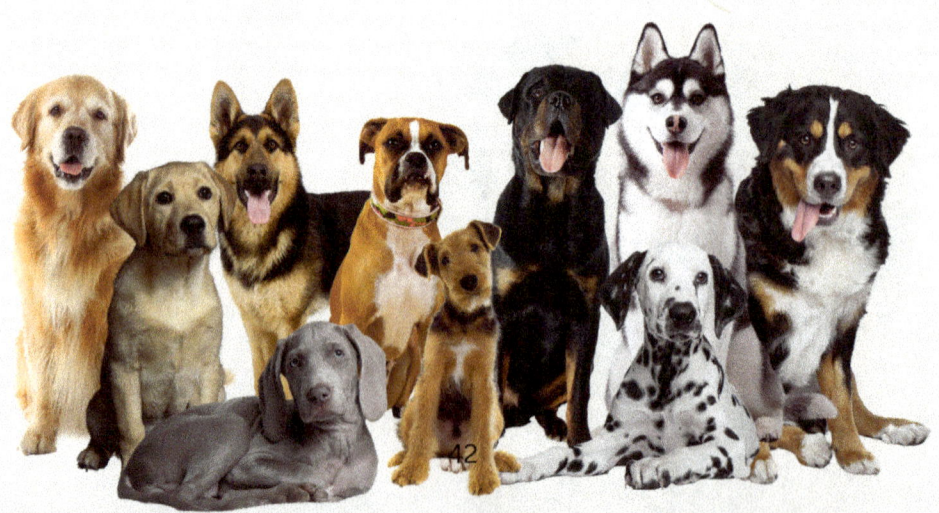

Signs of Hemoabdomen

- **Distended Abdomen:** A visibly swollen or enlarged abdomen is often the most noticeable sign.
- **Pale Gums:** This is often seen, especially if bleeding is happening rapidly. This indicates decreased blood circulation, which can be a sign of internal bleeding.
- **Weakness or Lethargy**: Your dog may appear unusually tired, lethargic, or unresponsive.
- **Rapid Breathing:** An increased respiratory rate occurs as the body tries to compensate for blood loss.
- **Abdominal Pain:** Signs of discomfort, such as flinching or guarding when the abdomen is touched, can indicate pain.
- **Vomiting or Retching:** These symptoms can suggest internal distress or irritation.
- **Behavioral Changes:** Increased agitation or restlessness may signal that your dog is not feeling well.
- **Collapse:** If hemoabdomen onset is rapid, the dog may acutely collapse.

Common Causes of Hemoabdomen

1. Splenic Tumors are the most common cause of hemoabdomen.
    a. The tumor can be due to a relatively benign cause, such as a hematoma in the spleen, but can also be due to cancers such as hemangioma and hemangiosarcoma (as well as some others).
2. Trauma: Physical injuries from accidents, falls, or fights can result in internal bleeding.
3. Clotting (Coagulation) Disorders: Conditions affecting blood clotting, such as exposure to rodenticide, von Willebrand disease, liver failure, or thrombocytopenia, can lead to spontaneous bleeding.

What Can You Do?

If you suspect your dog has a hemoabdomen, act quickly:
1. Seek Immediate Veterinary Care: Hemoabdomen is a serious condition that requires urgent evaluation and treatment by a veterinarian.
2. Avoid Manipulating the Abdomen: Do not press or poke your dog's abdomen as this can cause further pain or distress.
3. Keep Your Dog Calm: Try to keep your dog as calm and comfortable as possible while preparing for the vet visit.

Common Interventions:

Once at the veterinary clinic, the following treatments for hemoabdomen may occur:
1. Emergency Assessment and Testing: The veterinarian will perform a thorough physical examination and will recommend some blood work to evaluate the extent of blood loss and check organ function.
2. Imaging:
   a. Ultrasound: An abdominal ultrasound is often performed to visualize the source of the bleeding and assess for tumors or other abnormalities.
   b. X-rays: Radiographs may be used if ultrasound is not available or if there is concern for other causes for the bleeding.
3. Fluid Therapy: IV Fluids are often initiated to stabilize the dog, replenish lost fluids, and support blood pressure.
4. Transfusion: This may be needed, depending on degree of blood loss. This is often done at the time of surgery if bleeding is due to a ruptured tumor.
5. Surgical Intervention: In many cases, surgery is required to identify and address the source of bleeding, such as removing a tumor (e.g., splenectomy for splenic tumors).

Prevention

While not all cases of hemoabdomen can be prevented, you can take steps to reduce risks:
- Regular Vet Check-Ups: Routine veterinary visits can help identify underlying health issues, such as tumors or clotting disorders, before they become serious.
- Monitor for Signs of Illness: Be vigilant for any unusual behavior or physical changes in your dog and report them to your vet promptly.

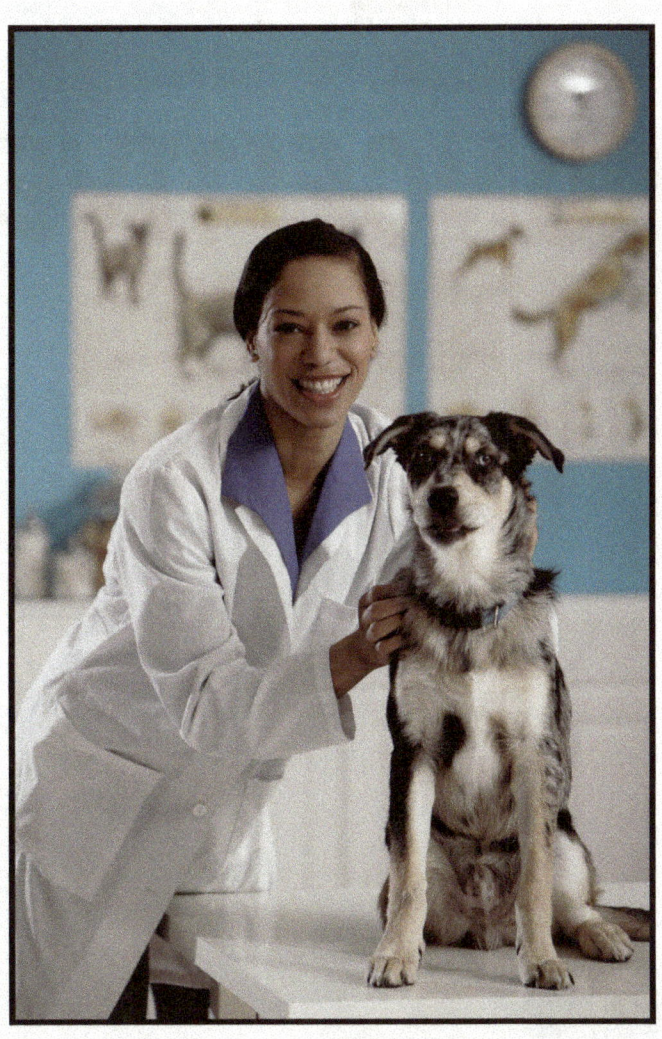

Emergency #8

CONGESTIVE HEART FAILURE

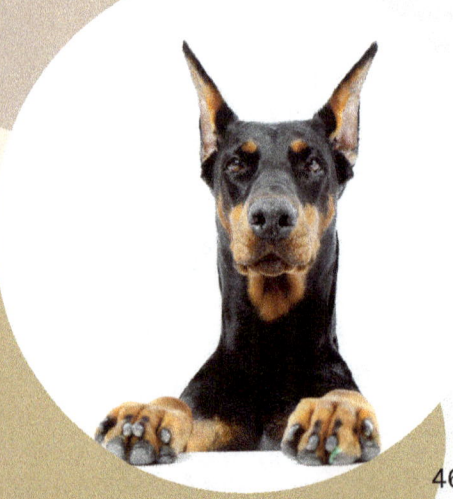

What is a Congestive Heart Failure (CHF)?

Congestive Heart Failure (CHF) is a serious condition that occurs when the heart cannot pump blood effectively, leading to a buildup of fluid in the lungs and other parts of the body. This condition often results from various underlying heart issues and is more common in older dogs.

Dogs Most Affected

Certain dog breeds are more predisposed to CHF due to genetic factors and specific heart conditions.

Some breeds commonly associated with a higher risk include the following:

1. Doberman Pinscher
2. Boxer
3. Cavalier King Charles Spaniel
4. Shetland Sheepdog
5. Golden Retriever
6. German Shepherd
7. Miniature Schnauzer
8. Poodle (Standard and Miniature)
9. Boston Terrier
10. Basset Hound

While these breeds are at higher risk, CHF can occur in any dog.

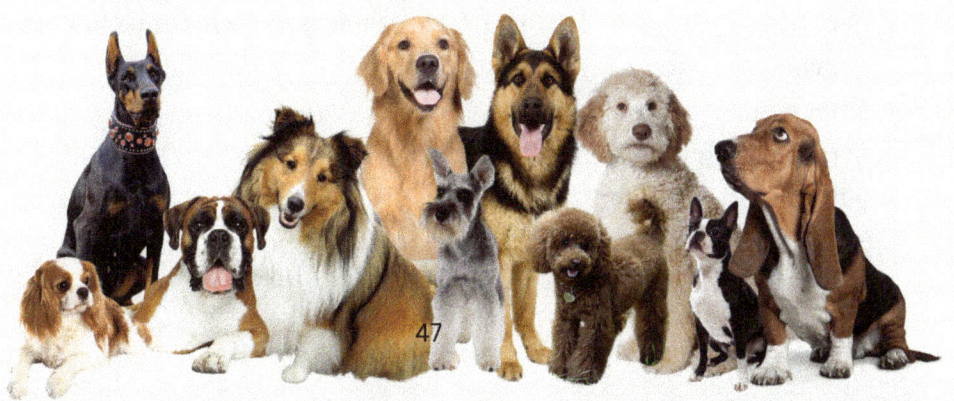

Signs of CHF

- **Coughing:** A persistent cough, especially after exercise or when lying down, is common in dogs with CHF.
- **Difficulty Breathing:** Increased respiratory rate, labored breathing, or open-mouth breathing may be apparent.
- **Lethargy:** Sluggishness, reduced energy, weakness, or lack of interest in normal activities may manifest.
- **Weakness/Collapse:** Fainting or collapsing (syncope), especially during exercise, may occur.
- **Fluid Buildup:** Swelling in the abdomen or legs (ascites or edema) may appear due to fluid accumulation.

Common Causes of CHF

There are many reasons why the heart may fail. Some causes are listed here:

1. <u>Dilated Cardiomyopathy (DCM):</u> This is a condition where the heart muscle becomes weakened and enlarged, leading to poor pumping ability. This is more common in larger breeds, such as Doberman Pinschers and Boxers.
2. <u>Mitral Valve Disease:</u> This is a degenerative condition affecting the heart's mitral valve, leading to blood leakage and heart enlargement. It is particularly common in small breeds like Cavalier King Charles Spaniels.
3. <u>Heartworm Disease:</u> This is a serious parasitic infection that can damage the heart and lungs, leading to heart failure if left untreated.
4. <u>Arrhythmias:</u> Irregular heartbeats can affect the heart's ability to pump effectively, contributing to CHF.
5. <u>Congenital Heart Defects:</u> Some dogs are born with structural heart defects that can lead to CHF.

What Can You Do?

Signs of CHF involve respiratory distress, which is a true emergency. Immediate care is needed.

1. Contact A Veterinarian: Contact your veterinarian or an emergency veterinarian immediately to let them know you are on your way. Ensure that the facility has the ability to provide oxygen support and hospitalization.
2. Keep Your Dog Calm: Minimize stress and allow your dog to rest while preparing for a vet visit.
3. Avoid Strenuous Activity: Keep your dog from engaging in excessive exercise, which can worsen symptoms.

Common Interventions:

At the veterinary clinic, the following treatments for CHF may occur:

1. Oxygen Therapy: Providing supplemental oxygen for dogs experiencing breathing difficulties is often needed.
2. Medications: Various medications are often needed during the initial stabilization process. These *may* include:
    a. Medication for anxiety: Dogs who can't breathe well are very stressed and this leads to worsening of their breathing.
    b. Diuretics can help to reduce fluid buildup in the lungs.
    c. Additional medications to improve heart contractility, relax the blood vessels, or manage heart rate/blood pressure may be needed.
3. Testing: X-rays of the chest are often recommended to assess severity and evaluate for other causes of breathing concerns. Blood work is often checked as well to assess overall stability.
4. Cardiologist Referral: As soon as the dog becomes stable, a cardiologist assessment will be recommended so as to perform an ultrasound of the heart (echocardiogram) as well as check pressures throughout the heart chambers and assist with long term therapy goals.

Prevention

CHF is likely not fully preventable, but there are some things we can do to try to lessen the likelihood of its development:

- **Weight Management:** Maintaining a healthy weight reduces stress on the heart.
- **Routine Checkups:** Yearly veterinary visits can help with early detection of a heart murmur and allow for extra monitoring and interventions prior to a crisis state.
- **Heartworm Prevention:** Regular testing and preventatives for heartworm will lessen or eliminate the possibility of contracting this disease.
- **Ensure a Healthy Diet:**
    - Avoid Grain-Free Diets: Recent studies have suggested a link between grain-free diets and an increased risk of DCM (Dilated cardiomyopathy), which may lead to CHF.
    - A balanced diet that includes all essential nutrients, including sufficient protein and taurine, is vital for heart health.

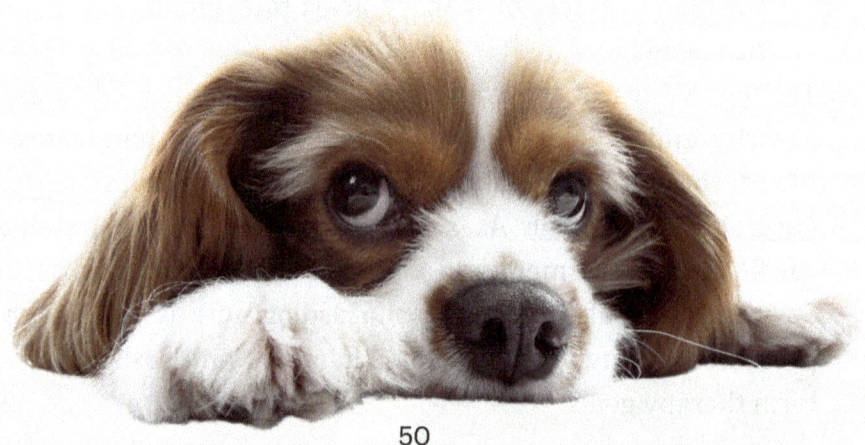

A Note About Oxygen Supplementation at the Veterinary Clinic

A dog who is struggling to breathe will often need to be taken to the hospital's treatment area to begin providing oxygen support.

There are several ways to administer oxygen.

Most of the time, this starts with an oxygen mask placed over your dog's face (See Fig 2.5, 2.6). This is a quick but temporary solution to provide oxygen, allowing the veterinary team to begin working with your pet as they gather additional information, such as placement of an IV catheter, drawing blood, and performing tests.

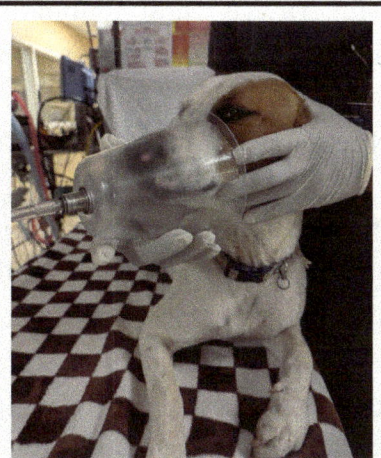

Figure 2.5. Image of a dog receiving oxygen support via an oxygen mask. This allows for the dog to remain accessible for the veterinary team, while providing the dog the oxygen they need.

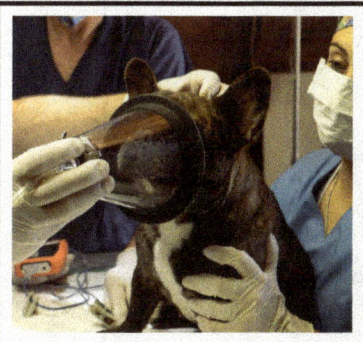

Figure 2.6. Another image of a dog receiving oxygen supplementation via a mask. Note that restraint is needed in order to provide support with this route. While this is OK for a short time period, it is not a good longer-term solution.

Dogs who arrive at the veterinary clinic with breathing difficulties will likely not be able to go home immediately. It takes time to resolve whatever issue has caused the breathing problems. Dogs are not likely to tolerate the oxygen mask for a prolonged time period and it does not allow them freedom of movement. Therefore, dogs are often moved into an oxygen kennel as soon as the veterinary team no longer needs to actively work with them.

The advantages of the oxygen kennel (See Fig 2.7) are numerous and dogs tend to respond very well to them. In the oxygen kennel, we can provide oxygen supplementation without needing to restrain or handle your pet. Additionally, we can control factors like temperature and humidity to ensure maximum comfort. Additionally, the white noise created by the machine and the enclosed environment help drown out the sounds of a busy emergency room, which can otherwise add to your dog's stress.

It's important to note that there may be times when visitation with your dog is discouraged while they are receiving oxygen support. This is particularly true for animals in severe distress who are also prone to anxiety or stress. When your dog is inside the oxygen kennel and sees you, they may focus their energy on trying to reunite with you. However, during times when breathing is difficult, it's essential that your dog focuses on one thing only - breathing.

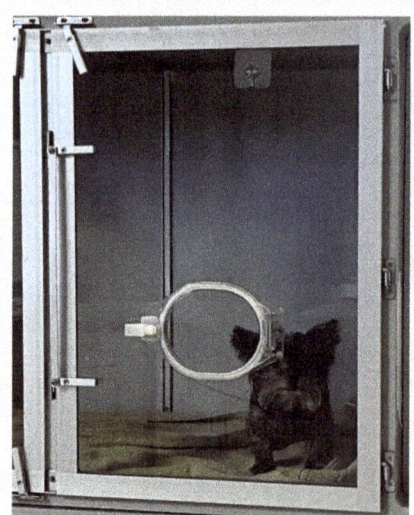

Figure 2.7. An image showing a dog who is within the oxygen kennel. The kennel is fully enclosed, allowing the dog freedom of movement within its space. The kennels regulate temperature and humidity and provide oxygen in a non-invasive manner.

Photo credit to Dr. Sara Thompson and "Maisie"

Emergency #9

VOMITING

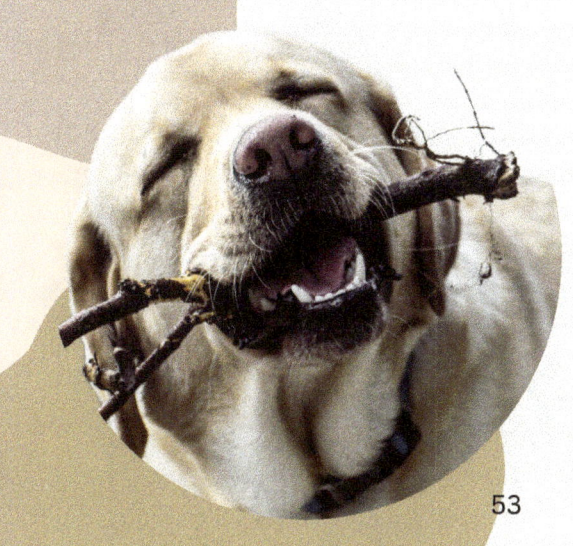

FOREIGN BODY

What is Vomiting due to a Foreign Body?

Vomiting is one of the most common reasons dogs visit the emergency room. While it can be triggered by something mild, like a change in diet, it can also signal more serious conditions such as parasites, systemic diseases, structural problems (like a foreign body), cancer, and more.

Since vomiting caused by a foreign object is particularly urgent and requires immediate veterinary attention, it will be discussed here.

Dogs Most Affected

Certain dog breeds are more prone to foreign body ingestion due to their behaviors, such as being overly curious or enthusiastic chewers.

Here are some breeds commonly predisposed to this issue:
1. Labrador Retriever
2. Golden Retriever
3. Beagle
4. Boxer
5. Bulldog
6. Cocker Spaniel
7. Dachshund
8. Border Collie
9. Jack Russell Terrier
10. Poodle

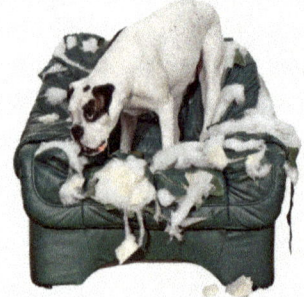

While these breeds may be more likely to ingest foreign objects, any dog can be at risk.

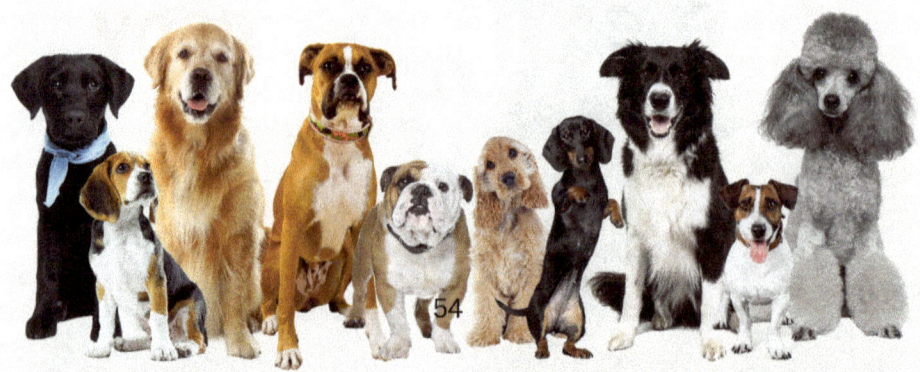

Common Materials Causing a Foreign Body Obstruction

There are many materials that dogs may ingest, which may fail to pass through the GI tract. Below are some common items.

1. Toys: Small parts of toys or entire toys can be swallowed, especially by enthusiastic chewers.
2. Clothing and Fabric: Dogs may chew and swallow pieces of clothing, blankets, or other fabrics, leading to blockages.
3. Food Items: Whole food items, like peach pits, corn on the cob, or food wrappers, can pose a risk if ingested.
4. Household Items: Objects such as rubber bands, string, or paper can be swallowed, causing gastrointestinal distress.
5. Natural Objects: Dogs may chew on sticks, rocks, or other debris during outdoor play, leading to ingestion.

Signs of a Possible Obstruction

- **Vomiting:** Frequent or persistent vomiting is the most common sign seen. At times the vomit may contain unusual objects, such as pieces of cloth, plastic, etc., which further increases the concern.
- **Loss of Appetite**: A refusal to eat or drink may be apparent.
- **Abdominal Discomfort**: Signs of pain, such as whining, pacing, or a tense abdomen may be seen, but are not always present.
- **Lethargy:** This is often seen, especially if the ingested item has been in the GI tract for some time.
- **Diarrhea:** Diarrhea, which may be accompanied by blood, may be seen, typically after vomiting has started.
- **Dehydration**: Signs such as dry gums, excessive panting, or lethargy may exist.
- **Weakness/Collapse:** If a foreign body is not identified and addressed, the bowel is at risk of perforating, and sepsis can ensue.

What Can You Do?

If you suspect your dog has ingested a foreign body, follow these steps:
- Contact A Veterinarian Immediately: Describe the situation, including what your dog may have ingested, the timeline, and any signs you may be observing.
   - The veterinarian will guide you with next steps, including potential at-home-care options.
- Do Not Induce Vomiting Without Veterinary Advice:
   - Inducing vomiting can sometimes cause more harm, depending on the type of foreign body.
- Keep Your Dog Calm: Minimize stress and allow your dog to rest while preparing for the vet visit.

If your dog is exhibiting concerning signs with ongoing vomiting, decreased appetite, etc., then a veterinary visit is warranted, whether you are aware of an ingested object or not.

Common Interventions:

If your pet recently ingested a foreign object of concern:
- Vomiting Induction may be an option, depending on the material ingested and the timeline. Your veterinarian will advise of this.

If your pet is vomiting and a foreign body is located:
- Veterinary Examination: A thorough examination to assess your dog's condition and determine if imaging (like X-rays or ultrasound) is needed.
- Endoscopy: In some cases, the vet may be able to remove the foreign body using an endoscope, which is a less invasive option.
- Surgery: If the foreign body cannot be removed via endoscopy or if there is a blockage, surgical intervention may be necessary.
- Supportive Care: This may include medications to manage vomiting and fluids to prevent dehydration.

Prevention

To help prevent foreign body ingestion, consider these tips:
- Supervise Playtime: Keep an eye on your dog when they are playing with toys or chewing items.
- Choose Safe Toys: Select durable, appropriately sized toys that are less likely to break into small pieces.
- Keep Hazardous Items Out of Reach: Store household items, food wrappers, and potentially dangerous objects in secure locations.
    - This is especially important and challenging with dogs who show an interest in ingesting fabric/ clothing.
- Be especially careful with food items that can be problematic such as peach pits or corn cobs.

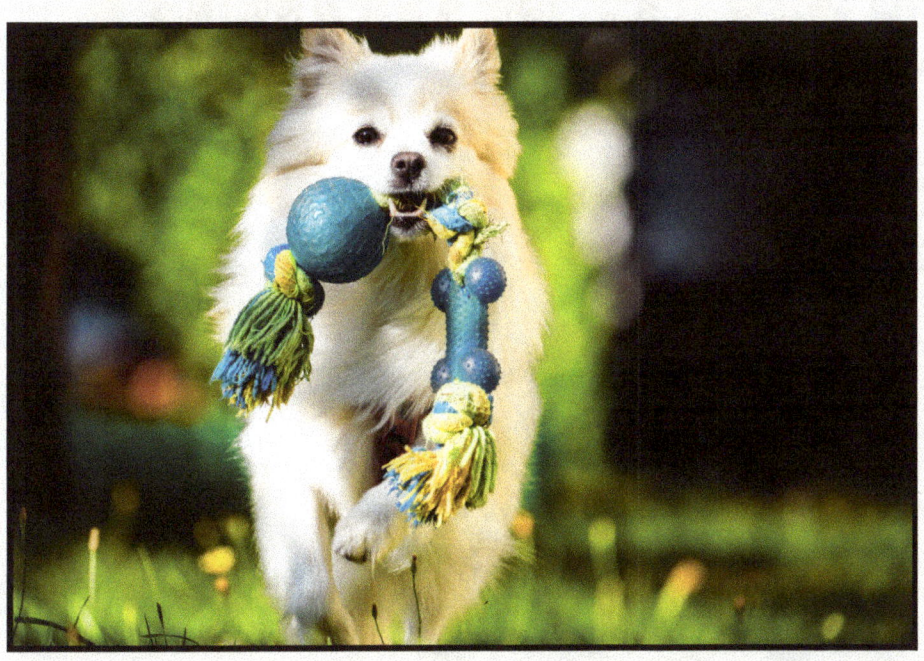

Emergency #10

BITE WOUNDS

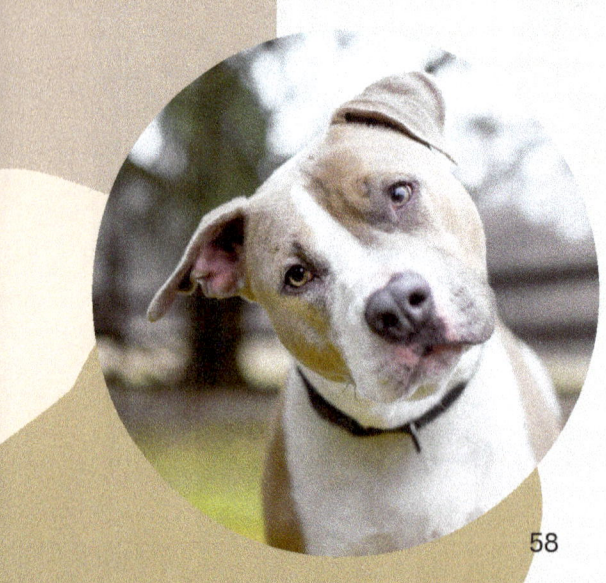

What are Bite Wounds?

Bite wounds in dogs can result from various sources, including fights with other animals, dog attacks, and encounters with wildlife. These wounds can range from superficial scratches to deep puncture wounds that may involve underlying tissues and organs, leading to serious complications.

Dogs Most Affected

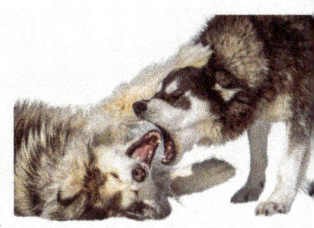

While any dog may sustain a bite wound, certain breeds may be more prone to situations that lead to bites due to their temperament, size, or socialization tendencies. Here are some breeds that may be predisposed:

1. **Pit Bull Terriers**: They are often involved in dog fights or aggressive encounters due to their strong prey drive and energy.
2. **Rottweilers:** Their protective nature can lead to aggressive behavior if they perceive a threat.
3. **German Shepherds:** Known for their guarding instincts, they may react aggressively in certain situations.
4. **Dachshunds:** Smaller size may lead to playful bites, especially during rough play with larger dogs.
5. **Chihuahuas:** Their small size can lead to aggressive behavior when threatened, resulting in bites.
6. **Boxers:** Playful and energetic, they can unintentionally cause bite wounds during rough play.
7. **Terriers**: Terrier breeds like Jack Russell and American Staffordshire have strong prey drives and can engage in fights with other animals.

Bite wounds can occur in any dog, regardless of breed. Factors such as lack of socialization, training, and environment play a significant role in a dog's behavior.

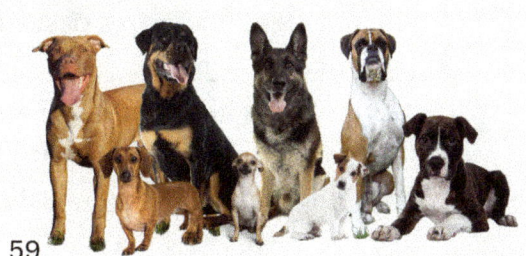

Signs of Bite Wounds

If your dog has sustained a bite wound, monitor for the following signs:

- **Visible Wounds:** Redness, swelling, or open wounds on the skin.
- **Bleeding:** Active bleeding from the wound site, which may be minimal or significant.
- **Pain or Discomfort**: Signs of pain, such as whining, yelping, or flinching when the area is touched.
- **Lethargy:** Unusual tiredness or reluctance to engage in normal activities.
- **Swelling:** Localized swelling around the bite area or throughout the body.
- **Foul Odor:** An unpleasant smell from the wound may indicate an infection.

The Golden Period

The "golden period" refers to the critical time frame following a bite wound during which prompt and appropriate treatment can significantly reduce the risk of infection and other complications.

This period typically lasts <u>no more than 6 hours</u> after the injury occurs.

1. <u>Infection Prevention:</u> The risk of bacterial infection is lower during the golden period, especially if the wound is cleaned and treated quickly.
2. <u>Wound Healing:</u> Prompt treatment facilitates better healing outcomes and minimizes tissue damage.
3. <u>Reduction of Complications:</u> Timely intervention helps prevent complications like abscess formation and systemic infections.
4. <u>Better Outcomes:</u> Dogs treated within the golden period are likely to require less intensive treatment and have shorter recovery times.

What Happens After the Golden Period?

Once the Golden Period has passed with a wound having not been addressed, we may be dealing with the following:
- Increased Risk of Infection: After the golden period, the risk of infection rises sharply.
- More Intensive Treatment Required: Delayed treatment may necessitate more aggressive interventions, like surgery.
- Longer Recovery Time: If an infection occurs, healing can be prolonged, requiring extended medication and follow-up visits.
- Increased Cost: Often times, the follow up and care that is required to deal with a wound that is no longer fresh leads to increased costs from what they would have been if addressed immediately.

What Can You Do?

If your dog has a bite wound, take the following steps:
1. Control Bleeding: If the wound is bleeding, apply gentle pressure with a clean cloth or gauze to control the bleeding.
2. Keep Your Dog Calm: Minimize stress and prevent your dog from licking or biting at the wound.
3. Contact Your Veterinarian: Describe the situation and follow their advice regarding the next steps.

Common Interventions:

Treatment of bite wounds may include:
1. Wound Cleaning: Professional cleaning may prevent infection.
2. Stitches or Sutures: Deep wounds may require stitches, but many bite wounds are left partially open to avoid trapping bacteria.
3. Medications: Antibiotics can prevent or treat infection and pain relief medications may manage discomfort.
4. Follow-Up Care: Regular check-ups are helpful to monitor healing and ensure no complications arise.

Prevention

To help prevent bite wounds, consider these tips:
- <u>Supervise Interactions:</u> Always supervise your dog during playtime with other animals.
- <u>Socialization:</u> Ensure your dog is well-socialized early to reduce aggressive behavior.
- <u>Avoid Common Triggers</u>: Do not have things like food or preferred toys around while dogs are playing.
- <u>Leash Control:</u> Keep your dog on a leash in unfamiliar environments to prevent encounters with wildlife or aggressive dogs.
- <u>Caution Around Challenging Areas:</u> Dog parks are a very common area where dogs often become injured.
  - This is partially due to overstimulation, resource competition, lack of full supervision, and multiple dogs with unknown temperaments in one area.
- <u>Ensure Up-to-Date Vaccinations:</u> Ensure your dog is up to date on their vaccines, especially rabies.

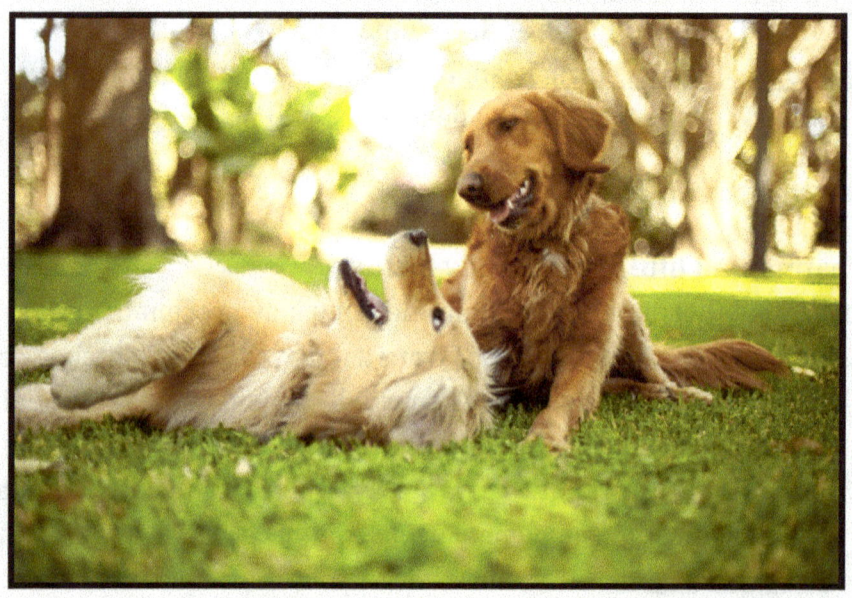

Chapter 3

TEN MOST COMMON TOXICITIES

With dogs' curious natures, exposure to toxic or potentially toxic substances is a common concern we see in veterinary medicine. While there are numerous possible toxicities, it helps to be familiar with the most common ones.

Upon evaluating 12 months of data collected by the ASPCA Poison Control in 2023, the top ten toxins will be discussed in this chapter.

Chapter Highlights

What to Do if Your Pet Ingests Something Toxic

Top 10 Toxicities:

1. Chocolate
2. Grapes/ Raisins
3. Xylitol
4. Bromethalin
5. Onions/ Garlic
6. Ibuprofen
7. THC
8. Vitamin D
9. Anti-Coagulant Rodenticide
10. Carprofen

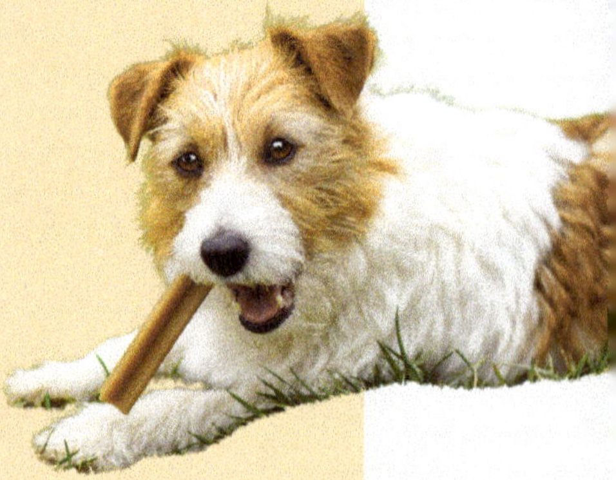

Note: Doses are generally calculated in mg/kg. That is the concentration of a medication/toxin in milligrams (mg) divided by the dog's weight in kilograms (kg).

To calculate your dog's weight in kg, simply divide their weight in pounds (lbs) by 2.2.
For example: a 22 pound dog / 2.2 = 10kg

ASPCA POISON CONTROL
(888) 426-4435

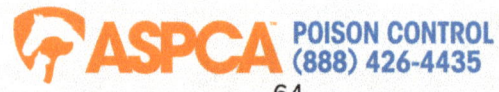

What to Do If Your Pet Ingests Something Toxic

- **Assess the situation and gather information.**
  - Identify **what** your dog ingested.
    - If you have the packaging available, have it handy.
  - Identify **how much** your dog ingested.
  - Identify **when** the dog ingested the product.
  - Have a rough idea of your dog's **weight**.
  - Keep track of any **clinical signs** you may be seeing.
- **Contact your veterinarian.**
  - For mild toxicities with known products, your vet may be able to provide sufficient guidance for the best way to ensure your dog's safety. However, be aware that a consultation with poison control may still be needed.
- **Contact Animal Poison Control.**
  - **ASPCA Poison Control:**
    - **(888) 426-4435**
    - Available 24/7
  - This service provides expert advice on what to do in any toxicity situation. They will discuss anything you can do at home, guide you through any procedure (like vomiting induction), or make recommendations for veterinary care.
  - They also provide guidance to any veterinarian who may be treating your dog.
  - You may opt to skip step 2 and call poison control directly!
- **Follow instructions** from your veterinarian/Poison Control.
  - Do not attempt to intervene at home without guidance.
  - Do not attempt to induce vomiting at home without consultation. In some situations, vomit induction will not be effective and can even be harmful.
- **DO NOT wait for symptoms to be seen**.
  - It is important to act immediately.
  - The earliest you begin interventions, the better the outcome.

Animal Poison Control Benefits

Some pet families are unclear about why we, as vets, recommend calling poison control for toxicities, as there is a fee associated with consultation. Here are some of the reasons why we do this:

- **Specialized Expertise**
    - Poison Control Centers are staffed by experts who specialize in toxicology and have access to extensive databases. They can provide the most accurate and up-to-date information regarding specific toxins and treatments.
- **24/7 Availability**
    - They operate around the clock, ensuring that pet owners can get immediate assistance at any time of day.
- **Follow-Up Care**
    - They are available for follow-up if any questions should arise about the situation in the near future.
- **Comprehensive Resources**
    - They have access to a wide range of resources and protocols that may not be available to individual veterinarians, allowing them to provide tailored advice based on the specific situation your pet is handling.
- **Guidance with Next Steps**
    - They help pet owners determine whether a situation is an emergency and what immediate action to take, including any home remedies or the need for vet care.
    - Guidance regarding care is also provided to any veterinarian who is caring for your pup.

Cost Effectiveness
- While there is a fee, the expertise and immediate guidance offered can save pet owners from costly treatments or missteps.

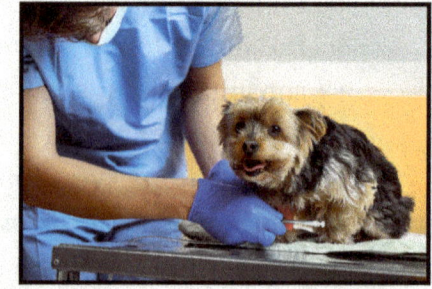

Toxicity #1

CHOCOLATE

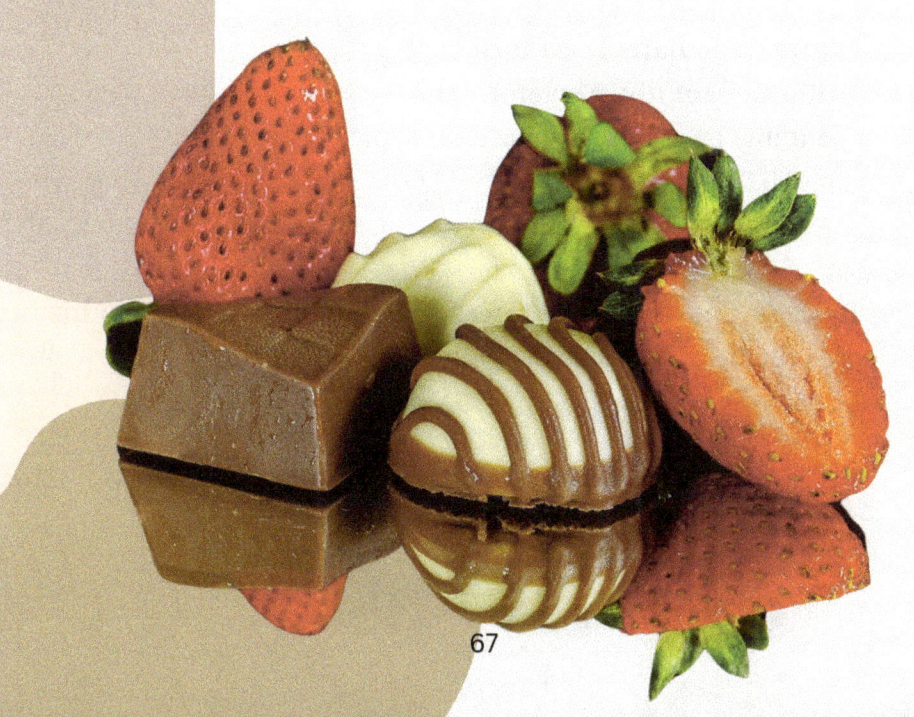

Chocolate is a common treat for humans, but it can be highly toxic to dogs. The primary toxins in chocolate are theobromine and caffeine, both of which belong to a class of compounds known as methylxanthines. Dogs metabolize these substances much more slowly than humans, making even small amounts of chocolate potentially dangerous.

Toxin: Theobromine and Caffeine

Theobromine is the main toxic component found in chocolate. Dark chocolate and baking chocolate contain much higher levels of theobromine compared to milk chocolate.

Caffeine is present in smaller amounts but also contributes to toxicity.

Both substances stimulate the central nervous system and cardiovascular system, leading to the toxic effects seen in dogs.

Toxicity Level of Common Chocolate Types:

MOST to LEAST

- **White Chocolate**: Least toxic
- **Milk Chocolate:** Moderate risk, which can be a concern depending on amount ingested. Typically, toxicities are seen around 0.5 ounces per pound.
- **Dark Chocolate:** Higher risk with toxic doses beginning at around 0.1 ounces per pound.
- **Baker's Chocolate** and **Cocoa Powder**: Very high risk; toxic doses can be at less than 0.1 ounces per pound.

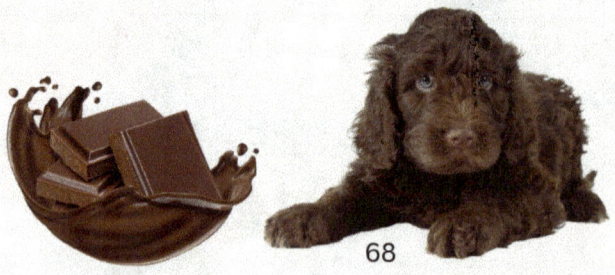

Symptoms of Toxicity

Symptom severity depends on the type and amount of chocolate ingested.

- Vomiting: This is one of the first signs as the body attempts to expel the toxic substance.
- Diarrhea: This often accompanies vomiting and can lead to dehydration.
- Hyperactivity/Agitation: This is commonly seen as the nervous system becomes stimulated.
- Rapid Breathing: Respiratory rate increases as the body struggles to cope with the toxin and the dog becomes agitated.
- Increased Heart Rate: Tachycardia can occur, leading to further complications.
- Seizures: In severe cases, neurological symptoms may arise, including seizures.
- Coma: In extreme cases of chocolate poisoning when veterinary intervention is not pursued, a dog may enter a state of coma.

Common Interventions at a Veterinary Facility:

If you suspect your dog has ingested chocolate, please seek veterinary assistance. Here are some interventions:
- Animal **Poison Control** should be contacted for guidance on severity of ingestion.
- **Interventions at a veterinary facility**:
    - Inducing Vomiting - depending on timeline
    - Activated Charcoal
    - Supportive Care - like IV fluids and medications to treat symptoms

Prognosis: With appropriate and rapid response, most dogs do well following chocolate ingestion.

Toxicity #2

GRAPES/ RAISINS

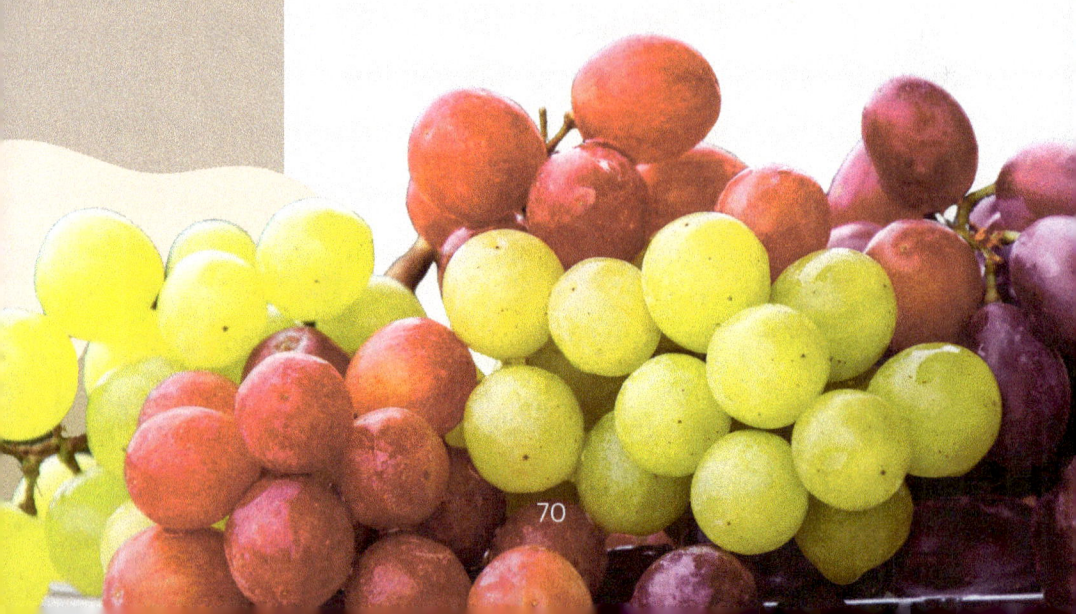

Grapes and raisins can be highly toxic to dogs. The specific toxic agent in grapes and raisins is not fully understood and not all dogs seem to be equally affected by ingesting the same amount. Even just a few grapes or raisins can lead to kidney failure.

Toxin: Tartaric acid and possibly others

The exact toxin in grapes and raisins is not fully understood, though several hypotheses have been proposed. Recent research has shown that tartaric acid appears to be the primary toxic compound, although additional unidentified toxins may also play a role.

Toxicity Level

The exact dose of toxicity is still unknown and seems to be due to multiple factors. However, it is generally estimated that more than one grape per ten pounds of body weight can cause serious toxicity.

It is important to note that there have been no reports of toxicosis from ingestion of grape juice or jelly.

Symptoms of Toxicity

- **Initial Signs (within a few hours)**
    - Vomiting
    - Diarrhea
    - Lethargy
    - Loss of appetite

    Note: Delayed signs may be seen in the absence of early signs.
- **Delayed Signs (within 24 to 72 hours)**
    - Increased thirst and urination
    - Abdominal pain
    - Kidney failure

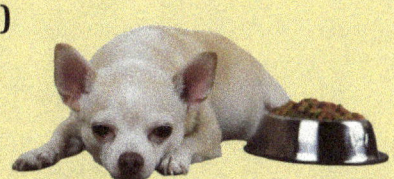

Common Interventions

- If the amount ingested is concerning, Animal Poison Control will generally recommend an immediate emergency visit.
- Common interventions at a veterinary facility may include:
    - Inducing Vomiting - to attempt to recover grapes/raisins
    - Administering Medications - to treat vomiting and settle the stomach
    - Providing IV Fluids - usually for at least 48 hours
    - Conducting Repeat Blood Work - to check kidney function, typically for at least 72 hours

Prognosis: With rapid intervention and absence of signs of kidney failure within 72 hours of ingestion, the prognosis is very good and it is unlikely that a problem will occur.

Prognosis becomes less favorable if kidney failure does occur.

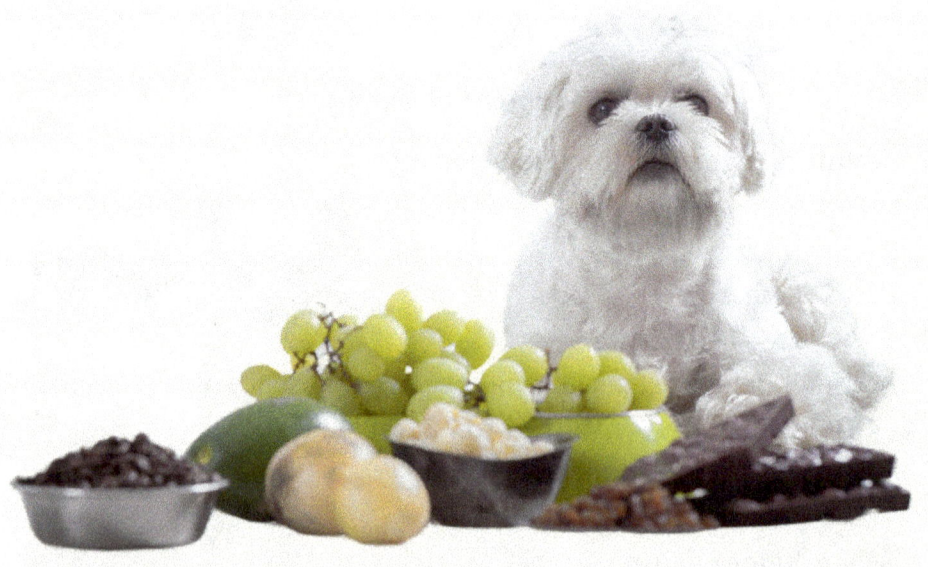

Toxicity #3

XYLITOL

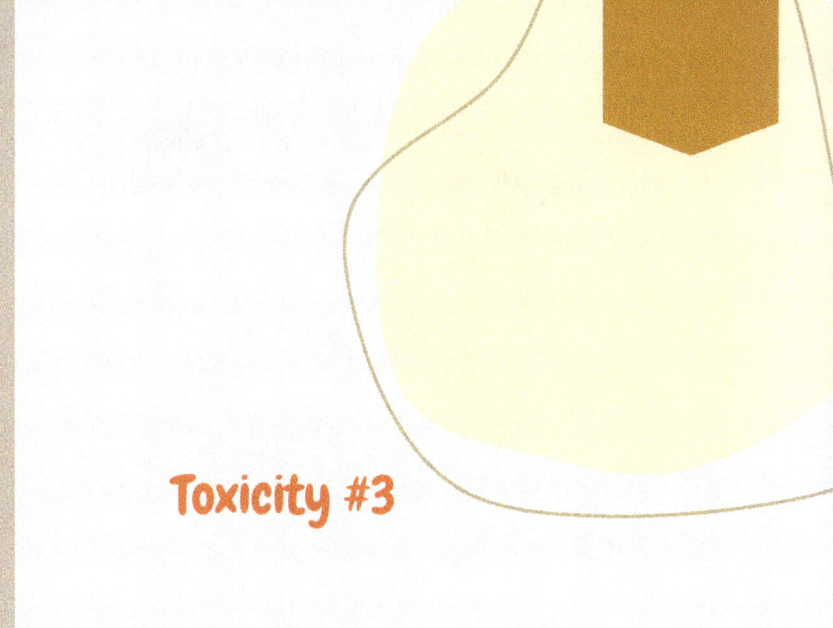

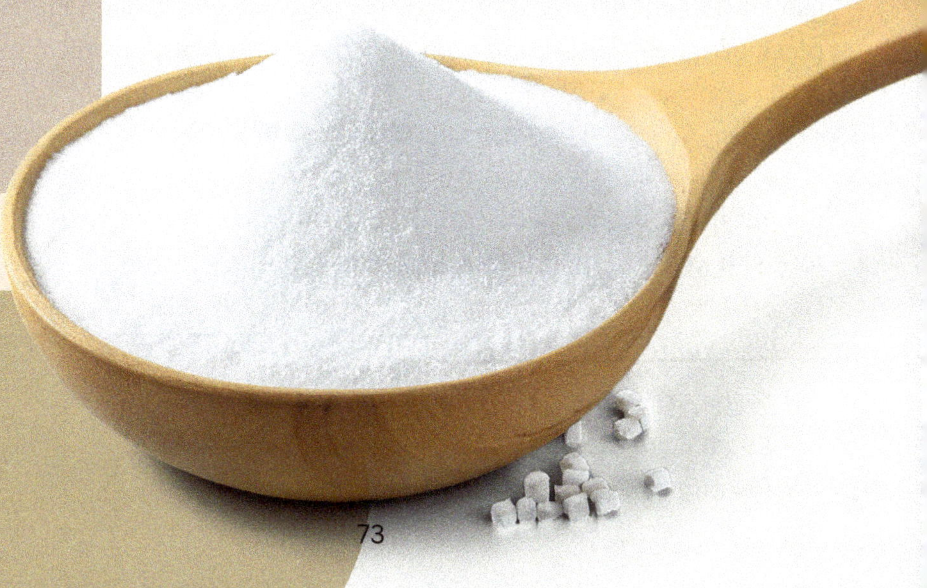

Xylitol is a sugar substitute commonly found in gum and other sugar-free products. It stimulates the pancreas to release insulin in dogs, which causes a rapid decrease in blood sugar levels (hypoglycemia). This insulin spike can occur even with small amounts of xylitol, leading to severe and potentially life-threatening consequences.

Toxin: Xylitol

Xylitol ingestion leads to an exaggerated stimulation of the pancreas, which results in a rapid depletion of stored body sugars and low blood sugar. The mechanism of causing liver failure is not fully understood.

Toxicity Level

Even a very small amount of xylitol can lead to severe reactions.
- Hypoglycemia: Signs can occur at doses less than 0.1 grams per kilogram (0.045g per pound) of body weight.
- Liver damage: Can occur at doses around 0.5 grams per kilogram (0.227g per pound).

For example: For a 10kg (22lb) dog, as little as one gram of xylitol can lead to clinical signs. Five grams can cause liver damage. A single piece of xylitol containing gum may have one gram of xylitol in it.

Common Causes/Sources of Xylitol

Labels must be checked closely if a dog ingested unknown human foods! If xylitol is listed as an ingredient, intervention is needed. **Be aware that xylitol may be listed as "Birch Sugar" on some labels.** Xylitol is found in:
- Sugar-free gum
- Sugar-free candy and baked goods
- Certain brands of peanut butter

Symptoms of Toxicity

The symptoms of xylitol poisoning can appear within 30 minutes of ingestion and may include:

- **Sudden Drop in Blood Sugar (Hypoglycemia)**: Hypoglycemia can lead to a range of symptoms such as weakness, lethargy, and disorientation.
- **Vomiting:** Dogs may vomit shortly after ingesting xylitol as their bodies react to the toxin.
- **Loss of Coordination:** Affected dogs may show signs of unsteadiness or difficulty walking.
- **Seizures:** In severe cases, hypoglycemia can trigger seizures.
- **Liver Failure:** Xylitol can lead to liver damage. Symptoms of liver failure may include jaundice (yellowing of the skin or eyes), increased bleeding tendency, and lethargy, which can occur several days after ingestion.

Common Interventions

Contact Animal Poison Control. They will likely recommend transportation to an emergency veterinarian.

- Common interventions at the veterinary facility may include:
    - Inducing Vomiting - although it may not be effective due to the speed of xylitol's absorption
    - Blood Sugar Monitoring - should begin at presentation and then every two to four hours
    - Liver Function Testing - begins at presentation and is then repeated
    - IV Fluids and Dextrose (Sugar Supplementation) - Even if the initial blood sugar is normal, dextrose supplementation is often administered to protect the liver.
    - Medications - administered to protect the liver and control symptoms
    - Hospitalization - a minimum of 12 hours is typically needed
    - Follow-Up Liver Tests - recommended until 72 hours after ingestion

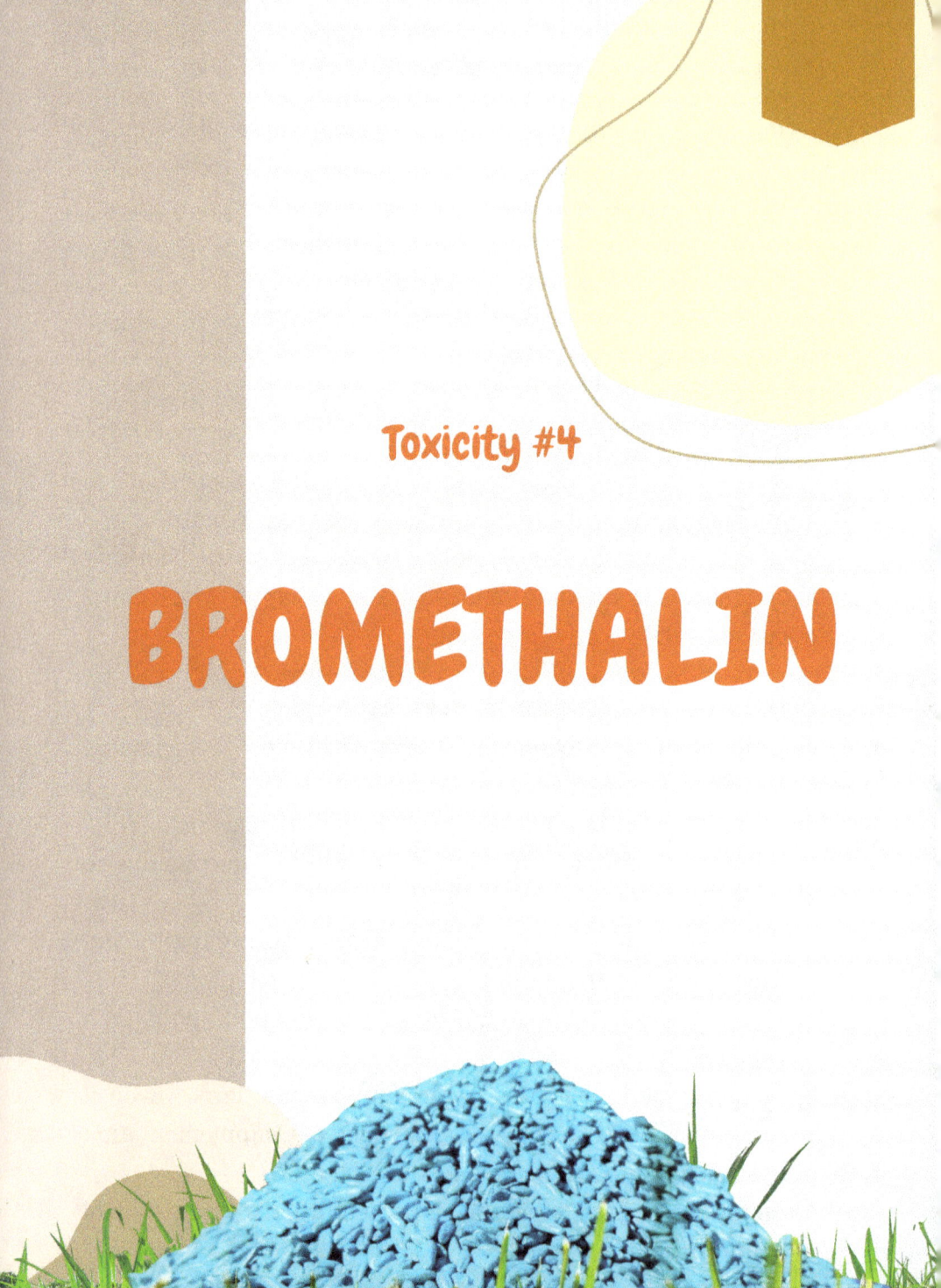

Toxicity #4

BROMETHALIN

Bromethalin is a type of rodenticide (rodent bait) that has become increasingly popular over the years. It is a neurotoxin, meaning it affects the nervous system of animals that ingest it, and it is highly dangerous to dogs.

Toxin: Bromethalin

Bromethalin affects the nervous system by disrupting the energy production in brain cells. This lack of energy leads to cell swelling and dysfunction.

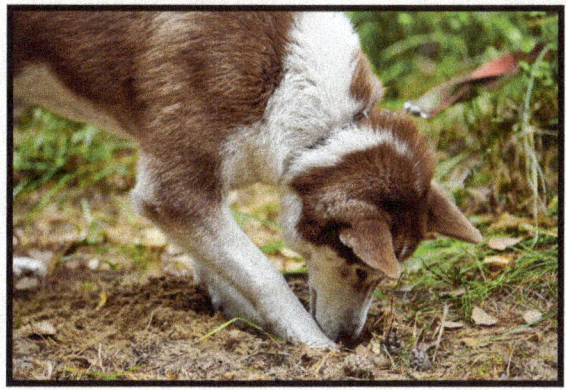

Toxicity Level

The onset of signs is variable, based on the amount ingested. Symptoms can appear within 12 hours of ingestion but may be delayed up to seven days.

The dose of concern is variable, but as little as 0.5 to 1mg/kg can cause serious side effects.

Unlike some rodenticides (rodent baits), this product does not have a direct antidote. As such, Animal Poison Control will recommend beginning decontamination and care at doses as low as 0.1mg/kg to prevent serious side effects.

Signs of Toxicity

Early Symptoms (within hours to days):
- Vomiting
- Loss of appetite
- Lethargy
- Tremors
- Seizures

Later (Delayed) Symptoms (within 24 hours to 5 days):
- Difficulty walking
- Muscle stiffness
- Coma or death

Common Interventions

- Call Animal Poison Control. This is essential!
    - It is vital to utilize the expertise of Poison Control to clarify the exact ingested dose and predict expected toxicities based on the product ingested.
- Common Interventions at a Veterinary Facility:
    - Inducing Vomiting - often recommended
    - Activated Charcoal - frequently used in multiple doses to continue binding the toxic principle in the stomach
    - IV Fluids and Symptomatic Care
    - Hospitalization - often required for a minimum of 24 hours

There is currently no antidote for Bromethalin toxicity.

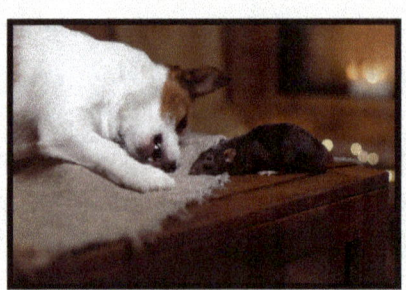

Toxicity #5

GARLIC/ ONION

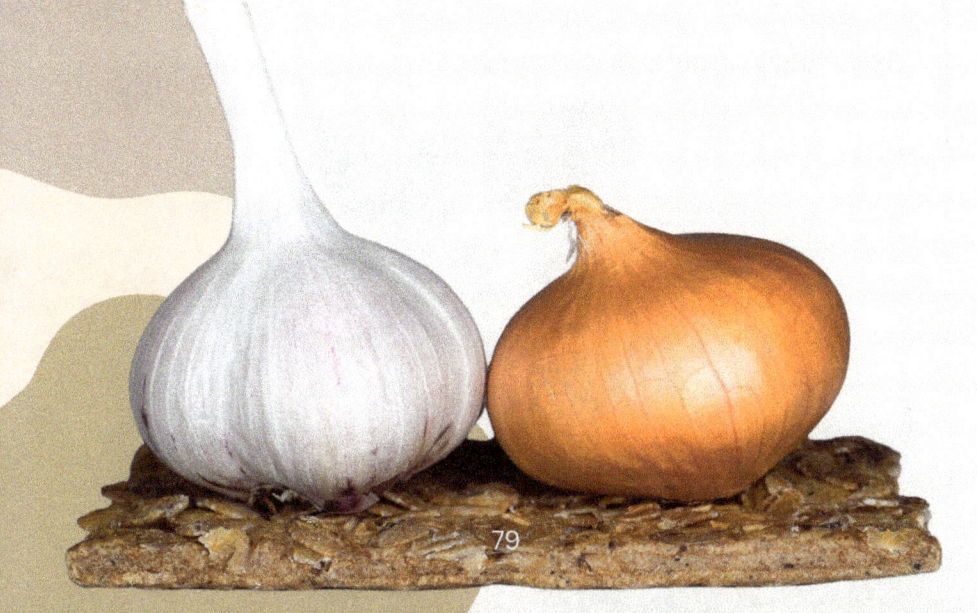

Common kitchen staples and garden vegetables like garlic and onions belong to the *Allium* family and contain toxins called disulfides, which can be harmful to dogs, leading to gastrointestinal signs and anemia.

Toxin: Disulfides

Disulfides can damage red blood cells, which may result in hemolytic anemia, where red blood cells are destroyed faster than they can be produced. Dogs lack certain enzymes that help protect their red blood cells from the effects of disulfides, making them particularly vulnerable to its toxic effects.

Toxicity Level

MOST to LEAST

- Cooked Onion: Least concentrated and not very toxic.
- Raw Onion: Mildly toxic. A fairly significant amount must be ingested before signs of concern appear. Usually, large chunks of raw onion are needed.
- Powdered Onion: More concentrated and thus more toxic, but typically a small amount is used in cooking.
- Garlic: Three times more concentrated than onions.

Toxicity may occur at 15g/kg of onions and 10g/kg of garlic.

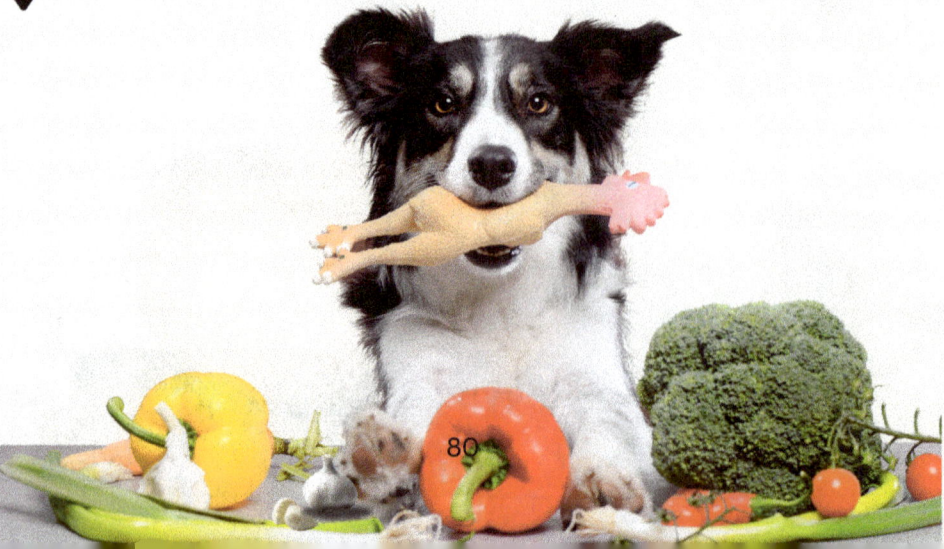

Symptoms of Toxicity

Symptoms of poisoning from onions, garlic, or chives may <u>not</u> appear immediately; they can take several days to manifest and may include:
- Vomiting: Dogs may vomit shortly after ingestion as their bodies react to the toxin.
- Diarrhea: This may accompany vomiting and can lead to dehydration.
- Lethargy: Affected dogs may show signs of weakness and a general lack of energy.
- **Decrease in Red Blood Cells (Anemia):** Symptoms of anemia may include:
  - Pale gums
  - Increased heart rate
  - Weakness
  - Collapse
  - Rapid breathing
  - Discoloration of urine
  - Jaundice

Common Interventions

- Contact Animal Poison Control for guidance.
  - At-home monitoring is often recommended.
- If a vet visit is recommended, common interventions may include:
  - Monitoring Blood Work
  - Supportive Care: Oxygen therapy and blood transfusions may be provided as needed until the body can make its own red cells again.
  - Red Blood Cell Monitoring: This will likely be recommended for about a week.

Toxicity #6

IBUPROFEN

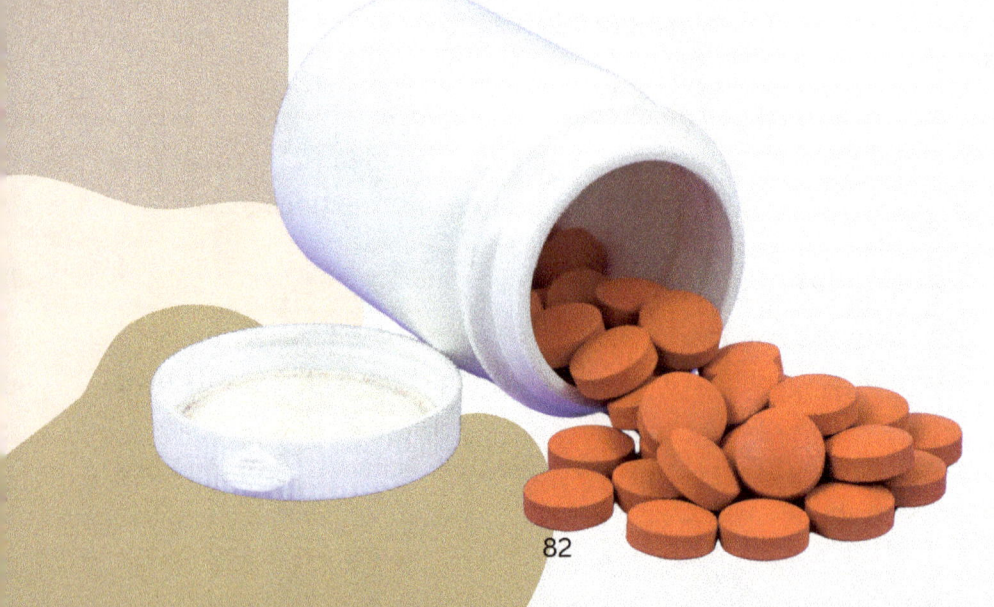

Ibuprofen is a common Non-Steroidal Anti-Inflammatory Drug (NSAID) used by humans to relieve pain and inflammation and is most commonly found in products like Advil and Motrin. However, it is toxic to dogs, and smaller dogs are especially at risk. The severity of signs can vary depending on the amount ingested.

Toxin: Ibuprofen

For dogs, the toxic agent in ibuprofen is the drug itself, which can cause gastrointestinal ulcers, kidney failure, and central nervous system issues, even at low doses.

Toxicity Level

- Gastrointestinal (GI) signs may be seen with ingestion of as little as 25 mg/kg.
- Stomach ulcerations are possible at around 50 mg/kg.
- Kidney failure may be seen at 125 mg/kg.
- Nervous system signs are possible with large ingestions, usually over 400 mg/kg.

Some animals will be more predisposed to the more serious side effects of an overdose. These include very small animals, older animals, or those with pre-existing kidney or liver diseases.

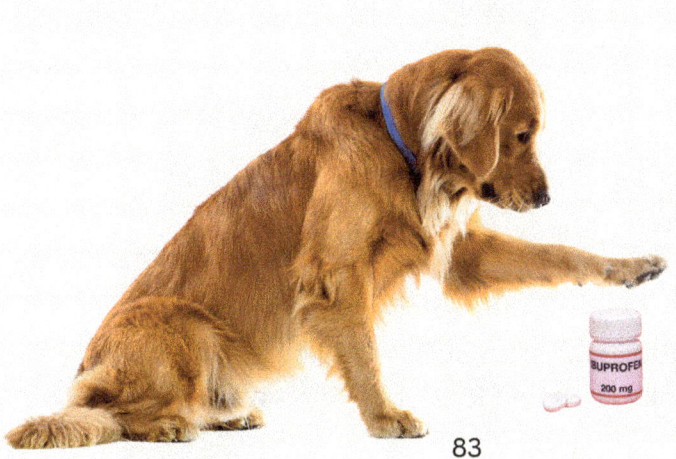

Symptoms of Toxicity

Signs are variable based on the amount of Ibuprofen ingested:
- Gastrointestinal (GI) Signs:
    - Vomiting
    - Diarrhea
    - Stomach pain/discomfort
    - Black, tarry stools
- Kidney Problems:
    - Increased thirst and urination
    - Lethargy
    - Kidney failure
- Nervous System Signs:
    - Uncoordinated movements
    - Seizures
    - Coma (at very large doses)

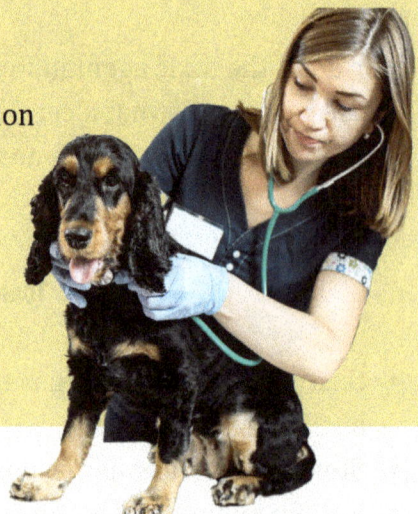

Common Interventions

- Animal Poison Control will assist you in determining whether the amount ingested is high enough to warrant emergency veterinary intervention.
- If a vet visit is recommended, common interventions may include the following:
    - Inducing Vomiting - depending on the timeline
    - Administering Activated Charcoal
    - Conducting Baseline Blood Work - especially to assess kidney values
    - Providing IV Fluids and Symptomatic Care - with medications to protect the gastrointestinal tract
    - Hospitalization - often for at least 48 hours
    - Ongoing Monitoring and Repeated Blood Work

Toxicity #7

THC

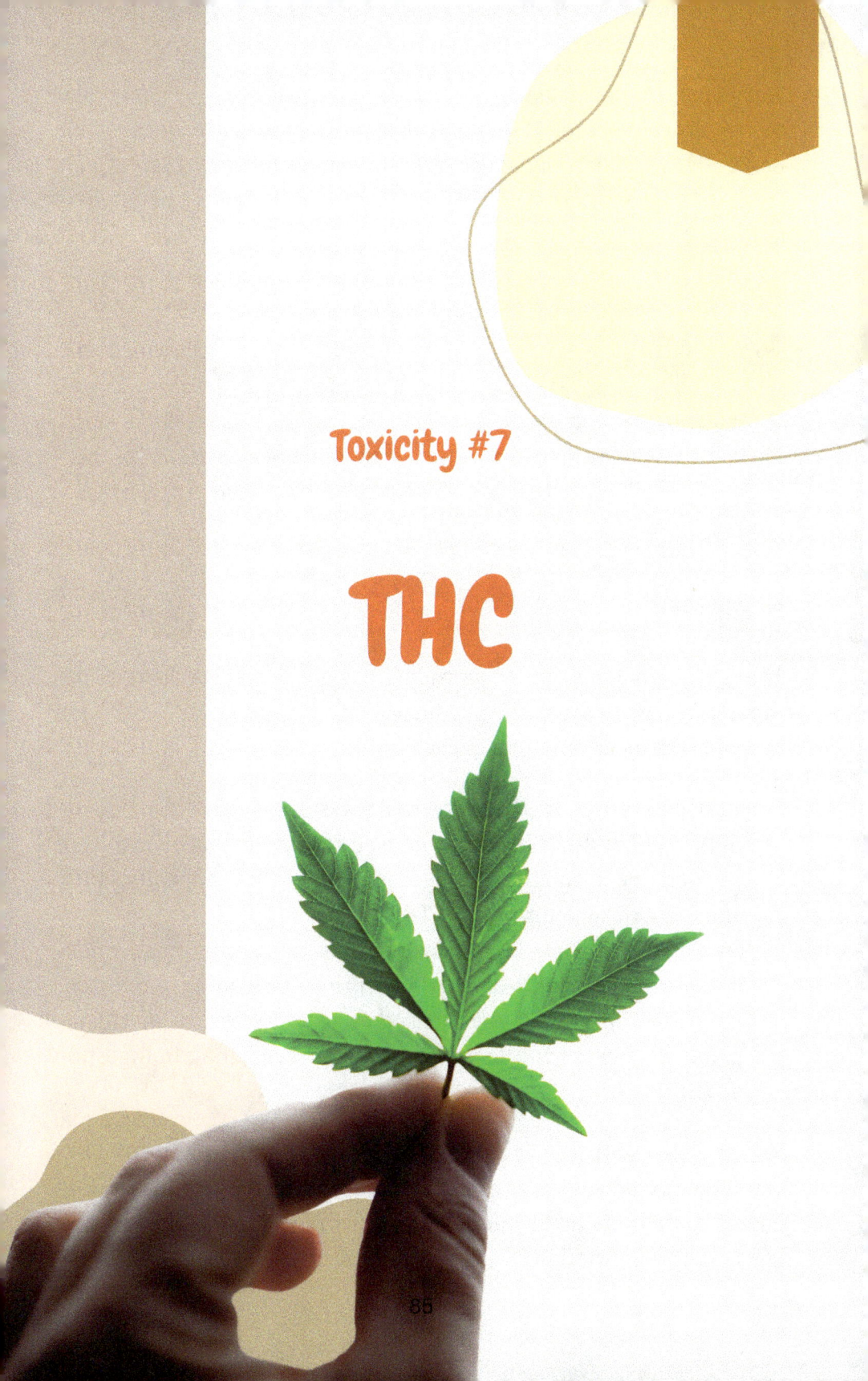

Marijuana, particularly its psychoactive component tetrahydrocannabinol (THC), poses significant risks to dogs. While perceptions of marijuana use are changing and it is increasingly legalized in many areas, it remains a serious concern for pet owners as dogs are particularly sensitive to THC.

Toxin: Tetrahydrocannabinol (THC)

THC affects the endocannabinoid system in dogs, which is involved in regulating various physiological processes. Dogs have a higher density of cannabinoid receptors in their brains compared to humans, making them more susceptible to the effects of THC. Even small amounts can lead to serious intoxication.

Toxicity Level

The toxic/lethal dose for this product has not been established. This is partially due to the many products available and lack of obligation to report the exact amounts in each product.

Dogs can be exposed to THC in several ways:
- Ingesting Edibles: Marijuana-infused foods, such as brownies or cookies, are particularly dangerous due to their appealing taste and higher concentrations of THC.
- Smoking Marijuana: Dogs may be exposed to secondhand smoke or consume remnants of marijuana products, leading to toxicity.
- Eating Marijuana Plants: Dogs that have access to marijuana plants may chew on the leaves or flowers, resulting in ingestion of THC.

Please Note: With the increase in popularity and legality of THC-containing products, many owners are unaware when their dogs have ingested this toxin (picked up outdoors, etc.) and present their dogs to the veterinarian due to the clinical signs seen.

Symptoms of Toxicity

Symptoms of marijuana poisoning can vary based on the amount ingested, the formulation, and the individual dog's sensitivity, but they typically include:
- Lethargy
- Sleepiness (somnolence): Dogs may fall asleep readily if not actively stimulated.
- Uncoordinated Movements
- Drooling
- Increased or Decreased Heart Rate
- Hypersensitivity to Stimuli (hyperesthesia)
  - Affected dogs often recoil with any stimuli near their face. This exaggerated motion is quite typical of THC intoxication and aids in diagnosis.
- Urine Dribbling
- Severe ingestions may lead to tremors, seizures, or coma.

Common Interventions

- Contact Animal Poison Control.
  - Fortunately, the vast majority of cases are self-limiting, meaning that dogs often do well without extensive intervention.
- If a veterinary visit is warranted, common interventions may include:
  - Administering subcutaneous fluids and anti-nausea medication.
    - Mild to moderate cases are often treated at home.
  - For significant toxicity, IV fluids may be recommended, along with supportive care until signs resolve. This typically lasts no more than 12-24 hours.

Toxicity #8

VITAMIN D

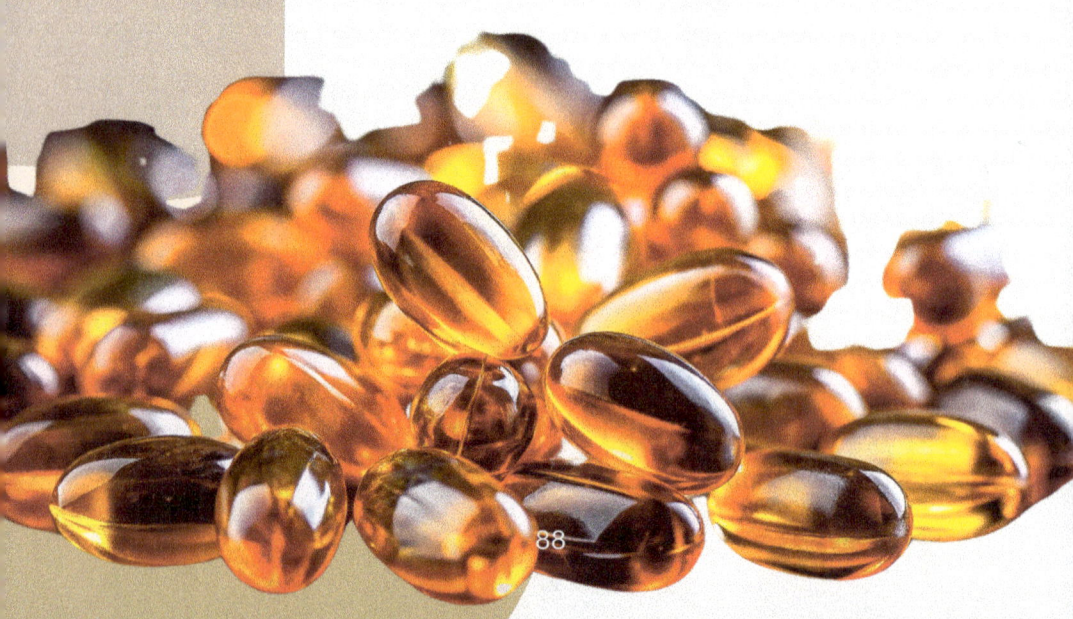

Vitamin D is essential for maintaining healthy bones and overall wellness in dogs. However, excessive ingestion can lead to toxicity, causing serious health issues. This can occur through accidental ingestion of Vitamin D supplements or through ingestion of Cholecalciferol rat bait (Vitamin D3).

Toxin: Vitamin D (Cholecalciferol)

Vitamin D promotes the absorption of calcium and phosphorus in the intestines. When ingested in large amounts, it can cause dangerously high levels of calcium in the blood (hypercalcemia), leading to calcium deposits in organs and tissues. Kidney failure is possible.

Toxicity Level

The toxic dose of cholecalciferol varies but can be as low as 0.1 mg/kg (=4,000 IU/kg). Clinical signs may develop within 24 to 48 hours after ingestion.

Other Vitamin D products have varying doses, depending on whether the product is Vitamin D2 or D3, as well as the size of the dog and diet they are being fed.

Poison control consultation is highly recommended for any ingestion of Vitamin D products.

Signs of Toxicity

Symptoms may take several hours to a few days to manifest. Key signs to monitor include:
- Early Symptoms (24-48 hours post-ingestion):
  - Vomiting
  - Loss of Appetite
  - Increased Thirst and Urination
- Progressive Symptoms (3-7 days post-ingestion):
  - Lethargy
  - Constipation
  - Abdominal Pain
  - Muscle Tremors or Weakness
  - Kidney Failure

Common Interventions

- Contact Animal Poison Control: Seek immediate guidance.
- Emergency veterinary care is often needed. Treatments include:
  - Inducing Vomiting
  - Activated Charcoal
  - IV Fluids
  - Monitoring Blood Work - especially calcium, phosphorus, and kidney values
    - often repeated daily for 4 days
  - Medications:
    - Cholestyramine reduces the absorption of cholecalciferol by directly binding it in the intestines.
    - usually prescribed for 4 days
  - Hospitalization need is variable based on amount ingested and the baseline bloodwork. Some animals are treated on an outpatient basis with daily repeated blood work.

Toxicity #9

RODENTICIDE

ANTI-COAGULANTS

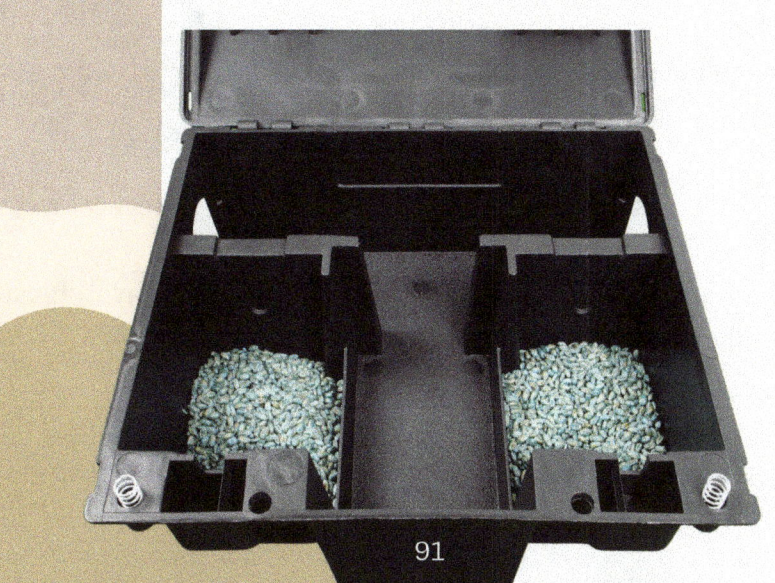

When a dog is exposed to an unknown rodenticide, the importance of calling Poison Control is amplified. They will have to consider ALL types of possible rodenticides in their calculations to assist with guidance. There are three main types of rodenticides, two of which have already been discussed (Bromethalin and Vitamin D). As a result, the focus here is on the third rodenticide: anti-coagulant rodenticide.

> **Toxin: Brodifacoum, Bromodiolone, and Difacinone**
>
> These rodenticides inhibit vitamin K recycling in the body, which is essential for producing clotting factors. Without adequate clotting factors, even minor injuries can lead to severe bleeding.

Toxicity Level

The toxic dose of rodenticide varies based on the product consumed and the amount ingested.
- Brodifacoum is most potent and has the longest duration of action.
    - Typically, expect signs at 0.1mg/kg.
- Bromodiolone is of medium potency.
    - Typically, signs occur at 0.5-1mg/kg.
- Diphacinone is the least potent.
    - Typically, signs occur at 1-2mg/kg.

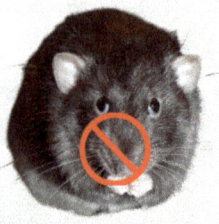

Dogs may be exposed to anticoagulant rodenticides in several ways:
- Ingesting Bait: Dogs may eat rodent bait directly.
- Eating Rodents: Dogs may consume rodents that have ingested the rodenticide.

Note: Signs are always going to be delayed with these products AND a direct antidote exists! Rapid action can lead to an excellent prognosis.

Signs of Toxicity

Symptoms of anticoagulant rodenticide poisoning <u>do not</u> appear immediately and can take several days to manifest.
- Initial Signs (1-2 days post-ingestion):
    - Lethargy
    - Loss of Appetite
- Later/Delayed Symptoms (3-7 days post-ingestion):
    - Pale Gums
    - Vomiting
    - Coughing or Difficulty Breathing
    - Abdominal Pain
    - Nasal Bleeding (Epistaxis)
    - Severe Weakness or Collapse

Common Interventions

- Contact Animal Poison Control: Immediate guidance is essential.
- If veterinary intervention is needed, common treatments include:
    - Inducing Vomiting: depending on timeline
    - Activated Charcoal
    - Vitamin K1 Therapy - administered to help restore normal clotting function; **this is a direct antidote!**
    - Blood Work - to monitor clotting factors and assess the extent of poisoning
    - IV Fluids - if ingestion was high
    - Hospitalization - may be required for severe cases, particularly if active bleeding is detected
    - Plasma Transfusion - if active bleeding exists

Note: With early detection and response, these dogs are often treated on an outpatient basis with Vitamin K1 administered at home!

Toxicity #10

CARPROFEN

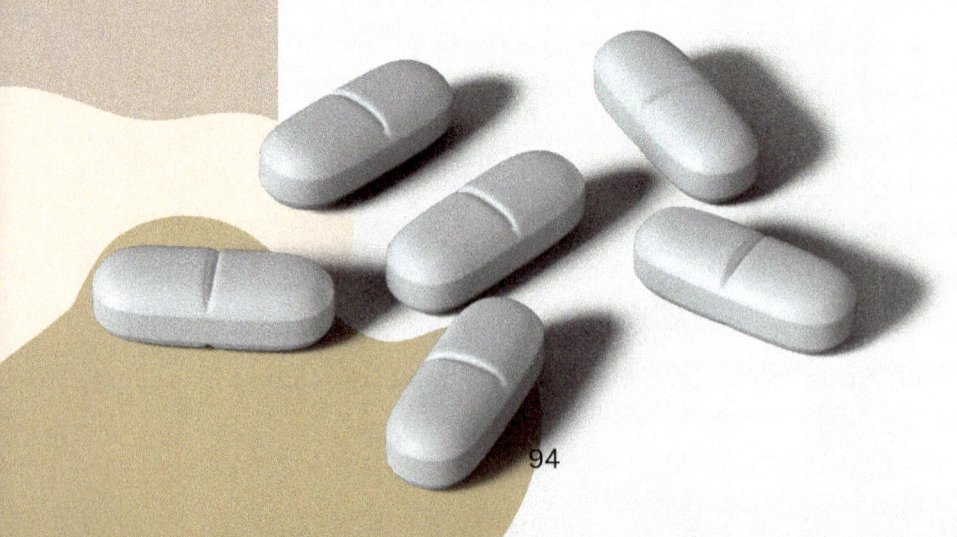

Carprofen is a non-steroidal anti-inflammatory drug (NSAID) commonly prescribed for dogs to relieve pain and inflammation. While carprofen can be highly effective, overdosage can lead to serious health risks. It is essential to adhere to the prescribed dosage and schedule provided by your veterinarian.

Toxin: Carprofen

The toxic agent in an overdose of carprofen for dogs is the drug itself, which can cause gastrointestinal ulcers, liver damage, and kidney failure.

Toxicity Level

The typical dose prescribed to a dog is no more than 4.4mg/kg.
- At a dose of 20 mg/kg:
  - Gastrointestinal effects may occur and may be profound.
  - These may include ulceration of the stomach/intestines.
- At 40 mg/kg:
  - Kidney failure may be seen.

Certain dogs are more susceptible to the toxic effects of an overdose. Those include smaller dogs, older dogs, or those with pre-existing kidney/liver disease.

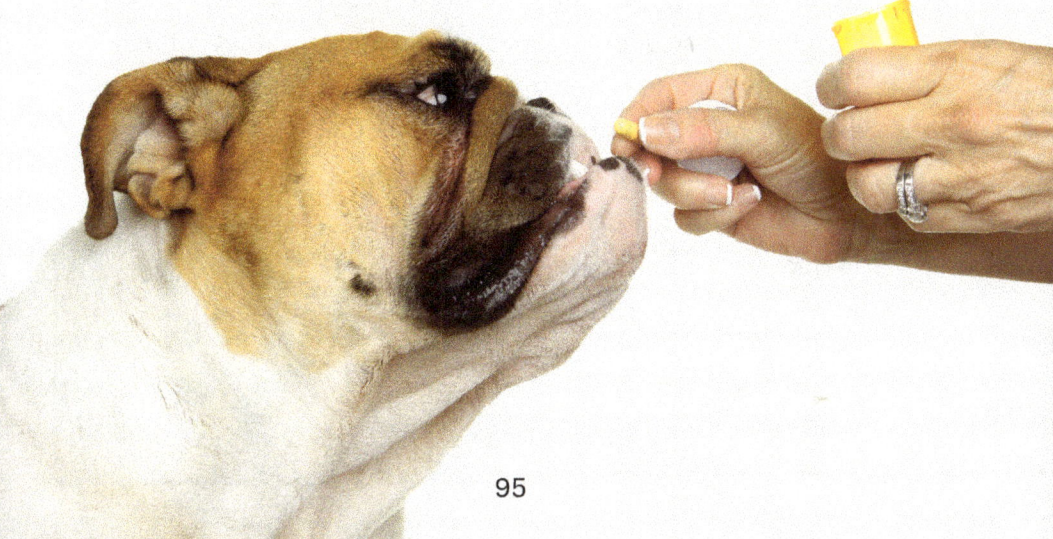

Signs of Toxicity

- Signs at lower toxicity doses:
    - Vomiting: may be repeated and severe
    - Diarrhea
    - Loss of Appetite
    - Lethargy
    - Abdominal Pain
- Signs at higher doses:
    - GI ulceration: blood in vomit/black stools
- Signs at doses high enough to cause kidney damage:
    - Increased Thirst and Urination
    - Increased severity of all the signs above

Common Interventions

- Contact Animal Poison Control. They will assist you in determining if the amount ingested is high enough to warrant emergency veterinary intervention.
- If a veterinary visit is recommended, common interventions may include:
    - Vomiting Induction
    - Activated Charcoal - may require repeated dosing
    - Baseline Blood Work - especially to assess kidney values
    - IV Fluids - along with symptomatic care and medications to protect the gastrointestinal tract
    - Hospitalization for 24-48 hours or more
    - Ongoing Monitoring - including repeated blood work

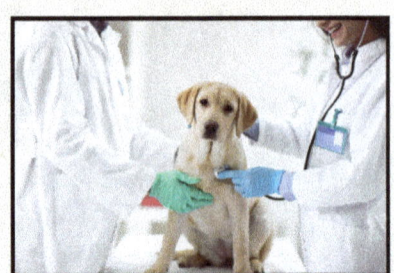

Chapter 4

HOW TO RECOGNIZE AN EMERGENCY

(COMMON SIGNS THAT OFTEN INDICATE AN EMERGENCY)

Determining whether your dog's symptoms are serious enough to warrant an emergency visit can be challenging. A helpful rule of thumb is this: If your dog is behaving unusually or showing signs of distress, it's wise to err on the side of caution. Contact your veterinarian or an emergency clinic for advice.

While minor issues like itchy skin, a mild upset stomach, or slight limping may not require urgent care, there are specific scenarios that demand immediate action. Below is a list of some common symptoms that should warrant a response by you. Sometimes this means asking your vet for advice. Other times, immediate evaluation by an urgent care or emergency (ER) veterinarian may be needed.

Chapter Highlights

Critical Signs that Should Not be Ignored:
1. Difficulty breathing
2. Severe vomiting and diarrhea
3. Sudden lethargy and weakness
4. Seizures
5. Bleeding
6. Severe trauma
7. Bloated/ distended belly
8. Sudden collapse/ unconsciousness
9. Severe pain/ difficulty moving

Subtle symptoms you shouldn't ignore

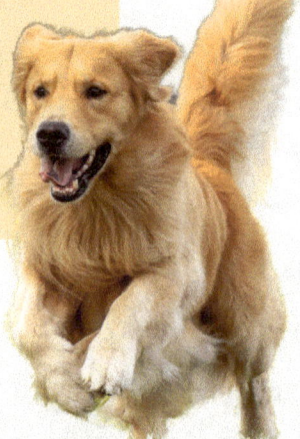

OVERVIEW

- Panting
- Respiratory effort
- Respiratory rate
- Accompanying signs of concern

True emergency!

DIFFICULTY BREATHING

SKILLS TOOLKIT

- Resting Respiratory Rate

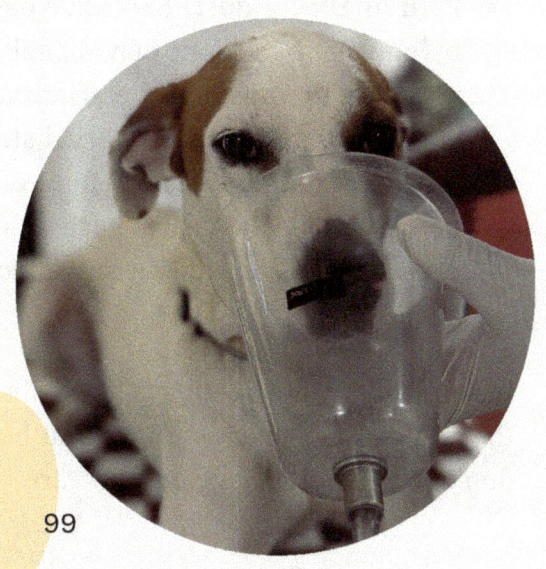

Breathing concerns can be confusing, making it hard to determine whether changes in your dog's breathing are normal or something to worry about. To identify what is abnormal, it's important to pay close attention to your dog's typical breathing patterns. Below are some guidelines to help you assess your dog's breathing and make an informed decision about urgency. Remember, if you're ever concerned, it's always best to seek care rather than delay.

Panting

Panting is a normal behavior for many dogs, but there are times it may indicate a concern. Here are some common reasons dogs pant:
- **Cooling Down:** Dogs don't sweat like humans; they regulate their temperature by panting. This evaporates moisture from their tongues and lungs, helping them cool down.
- **Exercise:** After physical activity, dogs often pant to bring their breathing rate back to normal and release excess heat.
- **Excitement**: Dogs may pant when they're excited or happy.
- **Stress or Anxiety:** Panting can indicate stress or anxiety, triggered by loud noises, new environments, separation from their owner, and more. If your dog frequently pants during stressful situations, consider discussing anxiety management with your vet.
- **Pain or Discomfort:** Excessive panting or panting accompanied by unusual behaviors may signal pain or illness. If this occurs, it's wise to consult a veterinarian, though it may not be an emergency unless respiratory distress is present.
- **Medical Conditions**: Persistent or unusual panting can indicate underlying health issues such as respiratory problems or heart conditions. If you notice any concerning signs, seek veterinary advice.

In summary, while panting is often normal, it's important to consider the context and your dog's overall behavior. If you have concerns, don't hesitate to seek veterinary care.

Respiratory Effort

Abdominal Contractions: Abdominal contractions can indicate respiratory distress in dogs. Normally, when a dog breathes, their chest expands and their belly rises slightly. However, if your dog's belly is moving in and out sharply or dramatically, it may signal trouble.

If you notice your dog's belly "heaving" or contracting tightly, it could mean they are not getting enough oxygen or are in pain. This is a serious concern that may require urgent veterinary care.

Difficulty breathing is medically referred to as dyspnea.

Respiratory Rate

Knowing your dog's normal respiratory rate is important for detecting breathing problems.

Resting Respiratory Rate (RRR): Monitor your dog's breathing while they are calm, not asleep.
- To determine the RRR, count the number of times their chest rises and falls in one minute. You can count for six seconds and multiply by ten to find the breaths per minute.

- Typically, a healthy dog's respiratory rate is fewer than 40 breaths per minute.
- Keep in mind that individual rates can vary. For example, a dog may breathe faster in hot weather. If you notice a consistent increase in your dog's breathing rate, it could be a cause for concern.
- Note: Do NOT count panting as an elevated respiratory rate unless other concerns also exist.

A rapid respiratory rate is known as tachypnea.

Signs that Accompany Respiratory Distress

When a dog is in respiratory distress, you may notice several accompanying changes in addition to increased respiratory rate and effort:

- **General Discomfort**: Signs include agitation, pacing, restlessness, and difficulty settling down.
- **Sleep Changes**: The dog may have trouble sleeping or may not be able to sleep at all.
- **Eating Habits:** Difficulty breathing can lead to poor eating or refusal of food as the dog focuses all its energy on breathing.
- **Neck Extension**: In severe cases, dogs may extend their necks forward, a position known as orthopnea, to help open their airways.
- **Respiratory Sounds:** You might hear coughing or wheezing, which can indicate the underlying cause of the distress.
- **Gum Color Changes:** Oxygen deprivation can cause gums to appear blue or purple (cyanosis) or pale due to poor circulation.

If you observe any of these signs, it's important to seek veterinary care.

Difficulty breathing, or dyspnea, is a serious condition that requires immediate attention. It's essential for pet owners to know their dog's normal breathing patterns to identify any abnormalities.

Monitor your dog's respiratory rate and effort and be aware of accompanying symptoms like lethargy, changes in appetite, or unusual behavior. Recognizing respiratory distress quickly can significantly impact your dog's health and well-being. If you're ever uncertain about your dog's breathing, consult a veterinarian promptly.

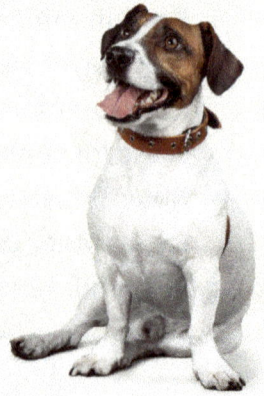

OVERVIEW

- Vomiting
- Diarrhea
- Signs of Dehydration
- Accompanying Signs of Concern

SKILLS TOOLKIT

- Gum Moisture Assessment
- Eye Assessment
- Skin Tenting
- Capillary Refill Times

True emergency!

SEVERE/PERSISTENT VOMITING/ DIARRHEA

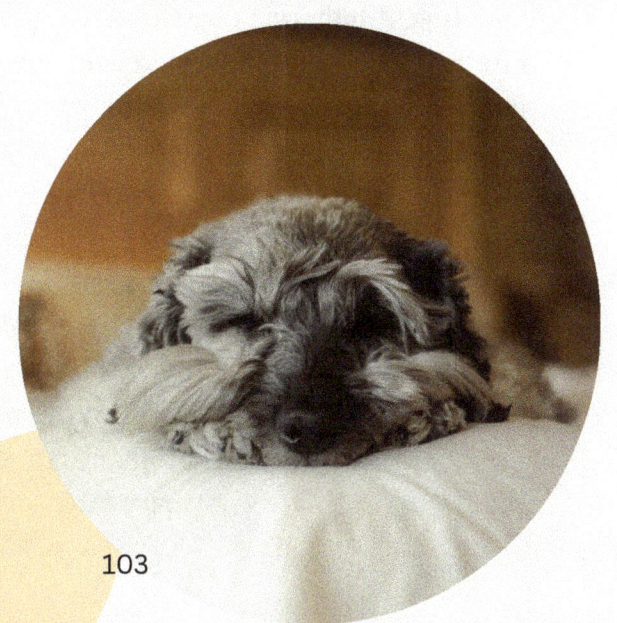

Vomiting and diarrhea are among the most common reasons pets visit the emergency clinic. While occasional vomiting or loose stools can be normal and are often due to dietary indiscretion or minor stomach upsets, persistent or severe gastrointestinal symptoms require immediate attention.

Because these issues are so common, it can be difficult for pet owners to know when to be concerned. As a general rule, if symptoms are persistent, worsening, or accompanied by behavior changes or blood, you should seek veterinary evaluation.

Persistent/ Frequent Vomiting

If your dog vomits more than two or three times in a 12-hour period, it may indicate the need for a veterinary assessment. Repeated vomiting can lead to **dehydration** and may signal a more serious issue, such as a systemic problem or obstruction. However, other behavioral changes should also be considered as they can provide additional insight into the severity of the situation.

Lethargy:
- Lethargy, or unusual fatigue, is often seen in conjunction with vomiting. A lethargic dog shows reduced energy levels, a lack of interest in normal activities, and may seem disengaged from family members. While some lethargy can occur naturally after vomiting, it is important to monitor your dog's behavior closely.
- Lethargy, especially when combined with vomiting, may indicate more serious issues such as dehydration, low blood pressure, low blood sugar, or even an underlying systemic problem.
- If your dog is still lethargic hours after vomiting and is not returning to normal activity, it is time to consult a veterinarian.
- If your dog is also unwilling to move, not interacting, or appears profoundly unwell, this is likely an emergency situation and requires immediate veterinary attention.

Lack of Appetite:
- A sudden refusal to eat after vomiting is not uncommon and is usually a protective response. However, this loss of appetite should not last for more than 24 hours.
- If your dog continues to show no interest in food or if there is a gradual decline in appetite over several days, this is a red flag.
- Dogs that fail to eat for extended periods can rapidly develop secondary issues, such as further dehydration or nutritional deficiencies, which can complicate the situation.

What About Acute Vomiting?

If your dog vomits once or twice and is otherwise acting normally with no signs of lethargy, the situation may be less urgent.

- A crucial factor to consider with acute vomiting is whether your dog was <u>fasted</u> after the vomiting occurred. *Many pet owners, with the best intentions, offer food or water right after vomiting, thinking it will prevent dehydration. However, this can often make the situation worse.*
    - When a dog vomits, their stomach becomes inflamed. Introducing food or water (or not restricting access to them) can further irritate the stomach and lead to <u>more</u> vomiting.
        - For this reason, we recommend withholding food and water for 6-8 hours after the first instance of vomiting.
        - For puppies and micro dogs, fast for 4-6hours.
    - If your dog has vomited only a few times and <u>is otherwise behaving normally</u>, try removing access to water for 6-8 hours to see if the vomiting subsides. If vomiting continues, it is likely time to seek veterinary care.

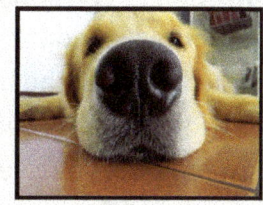

Persistent Diarrhea

Loose stools that last more than a few days, especially if they are <u>high volume, watery, or accompanied by blood</u>, may indicate the need for immediate veterinary care.

Diarrhea can quickly lead to dehydration, particularly in smaller dogs and puppies, so it's important to take these symptoms seriously.

Mild Diarrhea

In contrast, loose stools and mild diarrhea without discomfort or blood are often not emergencies and can typically be managed at home with dietary changes. If your dog has just started experiencing loose stools but is acting normally, consult your veterinarian to discuss dietary modifications as a first step.

Bland Diet Recommendations:
- **30% boiled lean meat** (e.g, ground turkey or chicken) and **70% low-fiber carbohydrates** (e.g, boiled pasta or white rice). Avoid salt, seasonings, or additives.
- Feed **small, frequent meals.**
- A general guideline is to feed <u>1 to 1.5 cups</u> of this diet <u>per 10lbs</u> of body weight, per day.

Additional Feeding Tips:
- **Fiber:** Adding canned pumpkin can help firm up stools by increasing the fiber content.
- **Probiotics**: Consider using veterinary-approved probiotics to support your dog's gut health.

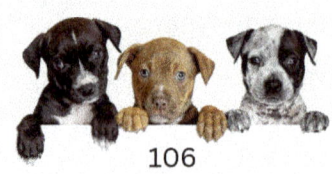

Signs of Dehydration

Dehydration can negatively impact various bodily functions. It's important to monitor for evidence of dehydration, especially if there's a known cause of fluid loss, like vomiting or diarrhea.

Below are some signs veterinarians use to assess hydration, which you can learn to check at home.

How to Check for Dehydration at Home

- Gum Color and Moisture:
    - Lift your dog's lip and examine the gums. Healthy gums should be pink and moist (See Fig 4.1).
    - If the gums feel dry or tacky, this may indicate dehydration.
        - Pale gums (See Fig 4.2) or severely reddened or purple (cyanotic) gums may be an indication of shock or further disease that requires immediate veterinary assessment.

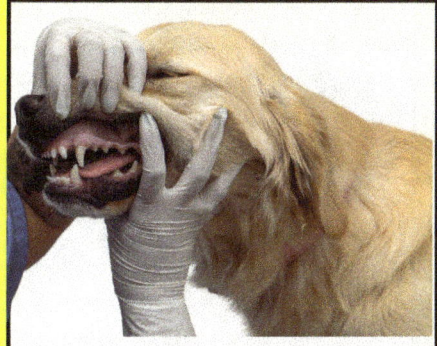

Figure 4.1: An image depicting a dog with normal pink gums

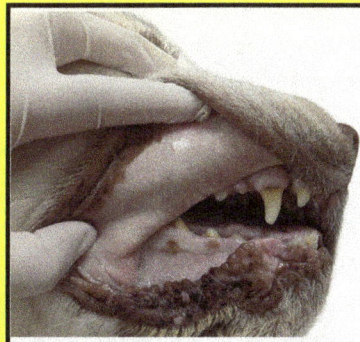

Figure 4.2: An image depicting a dog with pale and abnormal gums

- Assessing Eye Appearance:
    - Examine your dog's eyes. They should be bright, clear, and moist. Eyes should be comfortably seated in their sockets.
    - **Sunken** in or dull eyes may indicate dehydration.

- Capillary Refill Time (CRT) Test:
    - In a quiet environment, lift your dog's lip to expose the gums (See Fig 4.3).
    - Gently press on the gum area until it turns white (<1s) and then release.
        - Normal: Color returns in less than 2 seconds = good hydration.
        - **Prolonged (more than 2 seconds)** may indicate poor circulation or dehydration, which may require veterinary attention.
    - Tip: For dogs with pigmented gums, check the small pink areas around the teeth or on the underside of the lip for this test (See Fig 4.4).
- *CRT test explained: The CRT test measures how quickly blood returns to the capillaries after being temporarily pushed out. In a well-hydrated dog with adequate circulation and blood volume, blood will flow quickly to the gums and the color will return almost immediately. If your dog is dehydrated, the return of blood (and color) to the gums may be delayed.*

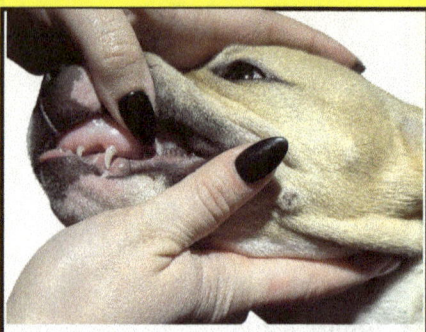

Figure 4.3. An image demonstrating positioning to check a Capillary Refill Time (CRT)

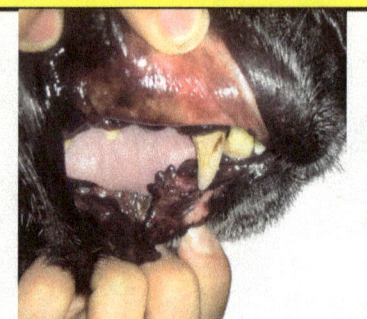

Figure 4.4. An image depicting a dog with pigmented gums. While the gums around the teeth will appear black, the underside of the lip is often pink and can be used to check gum color and CRT.

- Skin Tenting Test:
    - Gently pinch the skin on the back of your dog's neck or between the shoulder blades using your thumb and forefinger (See Fig 4.5).
    - Release the skin and observe how quickly it returns to normal.
        - Normal/Well-Hydrated: Skin returns to its normal position in <1 second
        - Mild Dehydration: 1-2 seconds to return to its normal position
        - **Longer than 2 seconds:** Moderate to severe dehydration is suggested, requiring immediate veterinary care.

Skin Tenting Explained: When dehydrated, your dog's skin loses moisture and elasticity. Healthy, well-hydrated dogs will have skin that is pliable and that snaps back into place immediately after being pinched. In dehydrated dogs, the skin will stay tented longer due to the loss of fluid.

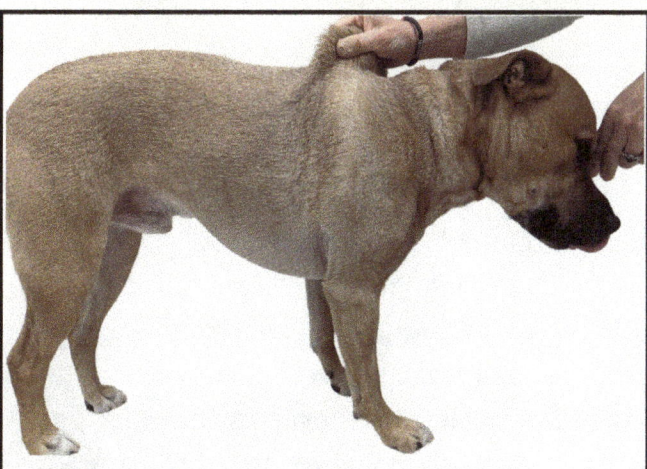

Figure 4.5. An image depicting the location and process of checking for skin tenting
Photo courtesy of Dr. Maria Bell and "Leo"

Checking for Dehydration At home: Practice

Checking your dog for dehydration may seem intimidating at first, but with a little practice, it becomes a simple process. Start by getting familiar with your dog's normal condition when they're healthy. This will make it easier to spot changes later.

1. **Check Gum Color:**
   a. Lift your dog's lips to examine their gums. Healthy gums should be <u>pink</u> (if not pigmented).
2. **Check Gum Moisture:**
   a. Rub your finger on the gums. They should feel <u>moist.</u>
3. **Capillary Refill Test:**
   a. Press gently on the gums to blanch them. Color should return in <u>less than 2 seconds</u> after releasing.
4. **Skin Tenting Test:**
   a. Gently pinch the skin on the back of the neck or between the shoulder blades. The skin should bounce back <u>immediately.</u>

With practice, you'll become comfortable checking these areas and can reassess them if you have concerns.

SUMMARY:

Severe or prolonged vomiting and diarrhea in dogs can be signs of serious underlying health problems that require immediate attention. By carefully monitoring your dog's symptoms and staying alert to signs of dehydration, lethargy, and other concerning behaviors, you can take swift action to protect their health. If you're ever unsure, it's always best to consult your veterinarian. Early intervention can make a significant difference in your dog's recovery and overall well-being.

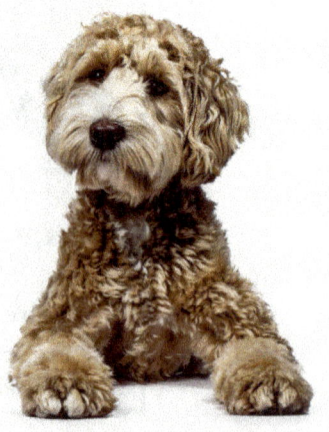

OVERVIEW
- Lethargy
- Weakness

True emergency!

SUDDEN/ PROFOUND LETHARGY/ WEAKNESS

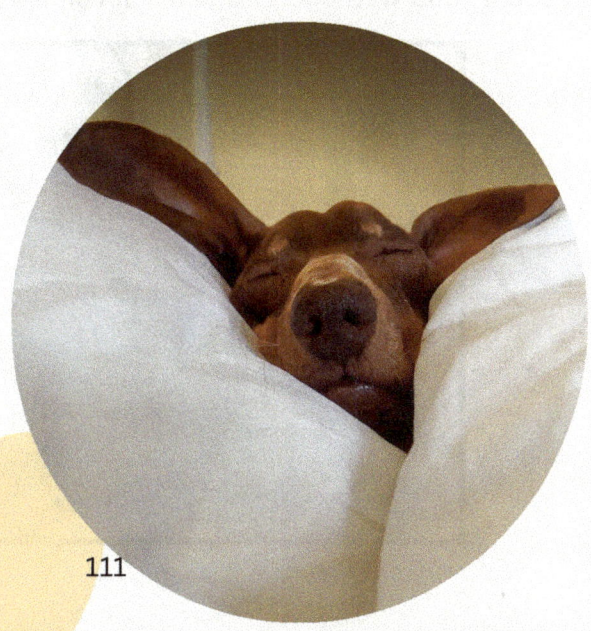

As a pet parent, it's essential to be familiar with your dog's usual behavior and energy levels. Dogs are naturally lively and curious, so any sudden change in their activity level can be a significant red flag. If you notice your dog becoming unusually lethargic or weak - such as refusing to stand, walking unsteadily, or even collapsing - this could signal a serious health issue that requires immediate veterinary attention.

Lethargy

Lethargy refers to a noticeable decrease in energy, causing your dog to seem unusually tired, sluggish, or weak. While some tiredness can be normal after play or exercise, sudden or persistent lethargy is concerning. It may be accompanied by other signs, like lack of appetite, difficulty moving, or reduced responsiveness.

Lethargy can be a symptom of various health conditions, from mild causes like stress or poor sleep, to more serious concerns such as infections, toxicities, or systemic illnesses.

Lethargy indicates that something is affecting your dog's overall energy and well-being - and it's not something to ignore.

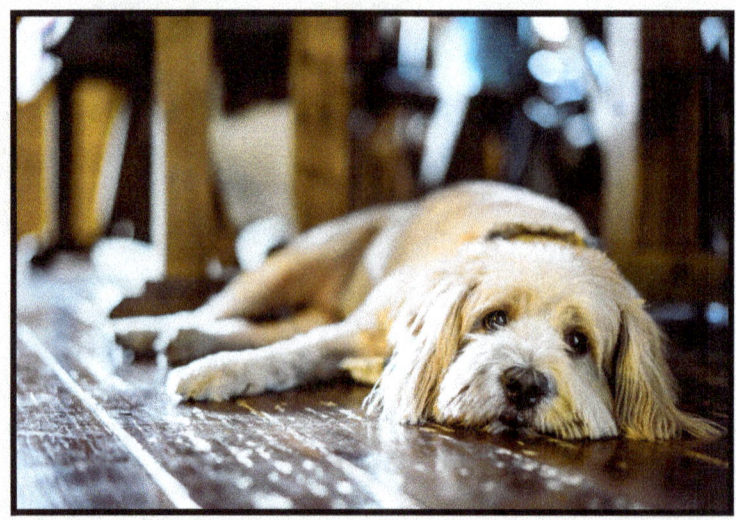

Signs Accompanying Lethargy, Increasing our Levels of Concern

Lethargy lasting more than 24hours:
- Lethargy, even if mild, that persists more than a day, should be evaluated by a veterinarian.
- Prolonged lethargy is not normal and could be a sign of a more serious underlying issue.

Refusal to stand or walk:
- If your dog is unwilling or unable to stand, this may indicate severe weakness or discomfort. This is particularly concerning if the reluctance to move is sudden or unexplained.

Poor responsiveness:
- If your dog isn't responding to you as they normally would - whether they don't react to their name, don't acknowledge commands, or seem disoriented - this suggests a problem that requires immediate attention.

Wobbly/unsteady gait/movement:
- General weakness can cause a dog to have trouble walking or balancing. If your dog's gait is unsteady or they're having difficulty moving and this is accompanied by other signs of lethargy, seek veterinary care right away.
- While changes in gait can be caused by orthopedic or neurological issues, when combined with lethargy, they may indicate a more serious concern.

SUMMARY:
Sudden lethargy or weakness in your dog is a serious concern that shouldn't be ignored. Recognizing these signs early can help you act quickly and reduce the risk of complications. Trust your instincts. If something feels off, seek veterinary help right away. Timely intervention can make a big difference in your dog's recovery.

OVERVIEW

- Grand mal
- Focal
- Seizure stages
- Determination of urgency

SKILLS TOOLKIT

- Seizure response

True emergency!

MULTIPLE/ PROLONGED SEIZURES

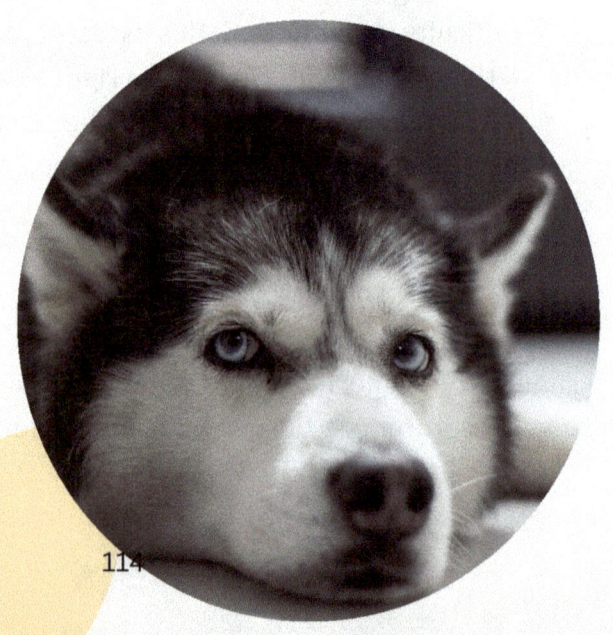

Seizures in dogs can be alarming for any pet parent. Understanding their nature and how to respond effectively is crucial.

Seizures are caused by abnormal firing of neurons in the brain. While grand mal seizures - characterized by full-body shaking - are the most recognized, other types of seizures exist. Not all seizures require immediate veterinary care, but knowing when to seek help is essential.

Types of Seizures:

Grand Mal Seizures
- These are the most common and recognizable seizures. During a grand mal seizure, your dog experiences body stiffness, collapse, muscle contractions, and paddling. They may lose consciousness and could also lose control of their bowels.

Focal Seizures (Partial Motor Seizures)
- Focal seizures affect only part of the dog's body and may or may not alter consciousness.
- Your dog may not lose consciousness, but may exhibit abnormal behaviors like disorientation, repetitive behaviors like "fly biting," or others.

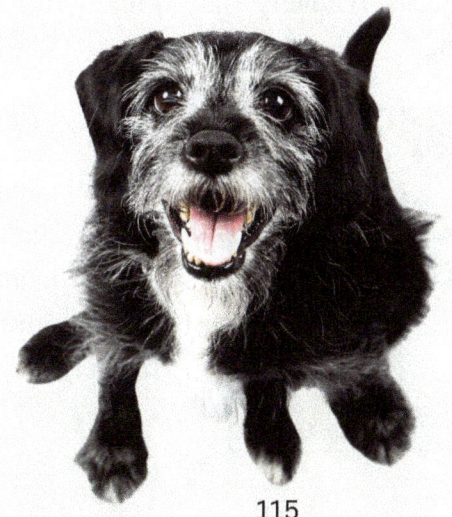

Seizure Phases:

Seizures can sometimes be confused with fainting spells caused by cardiovascular issues. A key difference is that seizures have **three** distinct phases:

1. **Pre-Seizure Phase** (Preictal)
   - This phase is subtle and varies from dog to dog. Signs can include restlessness, seeking attention, hiding, drooling, or agitation.
     - Being familiar with your dog's normal behavior will help you spot these early warning signs. However, you may not be able to recognize them unless your dog has had numerous seizures due to their subtle nature.
2. **Seizure Phase** (Ictal)
   - This is the active seizure phase, where neurological activity is at its peak. For a grand mal seizure, this typically involves body rigidity, convulsions, and loss of consciousness.
3. **Post-Seizure Phase** (Postictal)
   - After a seizure, dogs often appear disoriented, wobbly, or temporarily blind.
   - The postictal phase may last from minutes to hours and helps confirm a seizure event. This phase is distinct from syncope, where recovery is immediate and without disorientation.

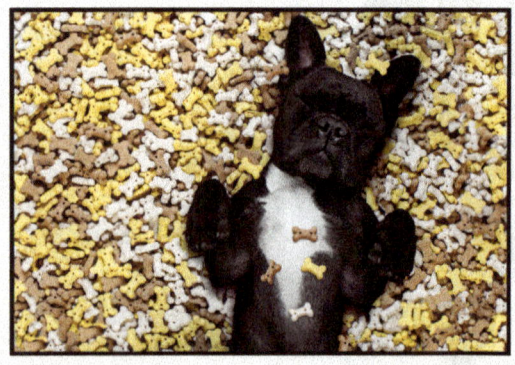

Many pet owners lump the postictal phase in with the seizure itself and, as a result, report pets having extremely long seizures.

What to Do if Your Dog Has a Seizure

1. **Ensure Your Dog's Safety**
   - Make sure your dog is in a safe area, away from stairs or sharp objects.
   - If possible, cushion their head with a pillow or soft material.
     - BE CAREFUL! Your dog will not have control of their movements and may bite!

2. **Time the Seizure**
   - Knowing how long the seizure lasts is valuable for your veterinarian. If the seizure lasts longer than three minutes, seek immediate veterinary care.
     - Remember - during a seizure, time may seem prolonged, so don't rely on your perception alone.

3. **Avoid Restraining Your Dog**
   - Do not try to hold your dog down or put your hands near their mouth. Dogs may bite unintentionally during a seizure.

4. **Observe and Record**
   - Take note of the duration and any unusual behaviors after the seizure, during the postictal phase. Recording this information can help your vet assess your dog's condition and treatment needs.

5. **Follow Up with Your Veterinarian**
   - Schedule an appointment with your veterinarian to discuss the seizure and determine the next steps. Keep in mind that while most single seizures are not emergencies, multiple seizures or additional symptoms require prompt attention.

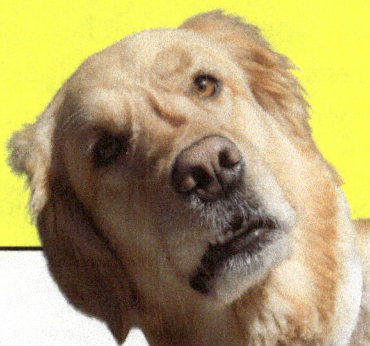

When are Seizures Emergencies?

All seizures warrant veterinary assessment. However, not all seizures are emergencies.

When Seizures Are a Priority - But Not an Emergency
A single, isolated seizure is not always urgent if:
- it lasts less than three minutes.
- the dog recovers fully and shows no lasting behavioral changes.

When Seizures Are an Emergency
Consider a seizure an emergency when:
- three or more seizures are noted in a 24-hour period.
- a single seizure is followed by prolonged lethargy, weakness, or significant behavioral changes.
- a seizure occurs in a dog who has other serious health concerns (e.g., not eating, weight loss, lethargy).
- seizures occur in very young puppies (under six months) or small dogs (under ten pounds).

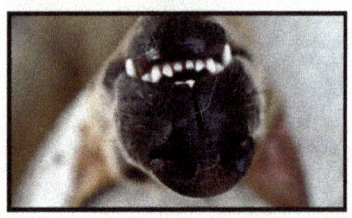

SUMMARY:
Seizures can be frightening but knowing how to recognize different types of seizures and how to respond can make a significant difference in your dog's well-being. While not every seizure requires emergency care, timely veterinary evaluation is essential, especially if seizures are frequent or accompanied by other concerning symptoms. Always trust your instincts and obtain veterinarian care if you are concerned.

OVERVIEW

- External bleeding
- Internal bleeding
- Signs of significant blood loss

SKILLS TOOLKIT

- Managing simple external bleeding

Possible emergency

BLEEDING

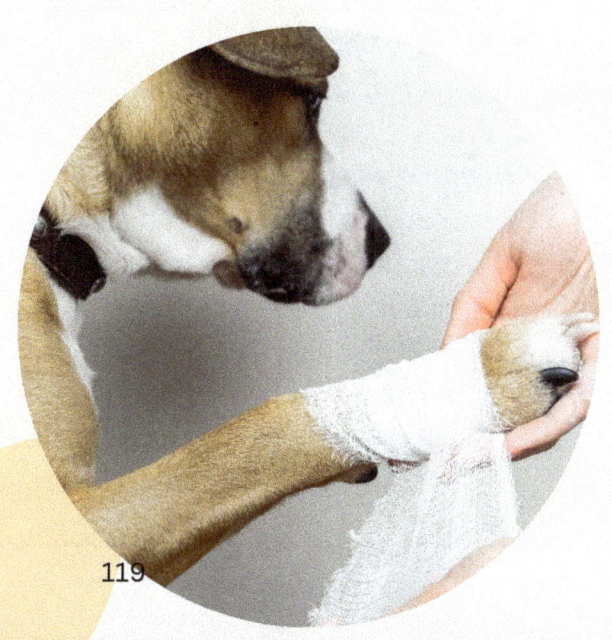

Bleeding, whether external or internal, can be a serious concern for your dog. While external bleeding can often be managed with proper first aid, internal bleeding may require immediate veterinary care. Let's break down the ways to recognize and respond to different types of bleeding.

Recognizing and Managing External and Internal Bleeding

EXTERNAL Bleeding

- External bleeding can often be controlled by applying direct pressure to the affected area.
- This is especially effective for smaller injuries, like small wounds or a toenail injury.

How to Manage External Bleeding

For minor wounds or toenail injuries:
- Apply pressure: Firm, consistent pressure is key to stopping the bleeding. Resist the urge to check too soon. Keep applying pressure for at least five minutes to allow a clot to form.
- Clotting aids:
  - For TOENAILS only: If bleeding persists, you can use baking soda, cornstarch, or baking powder to help form a clot.
- Note: Depending on the cause of the bleeding, veterinary care may still be needed, even if bleeding has stopped.
  - Wounds, for example, can easily become infected and require veterinary care much of the time.

INTERNAL Bleeding

Internal bleeding can occur after trauma, exposure to toxins (like rat poison), or due to certain medical conditions. Since the blood isn't visible, it's important to watch for signs of blood loss or anemia.

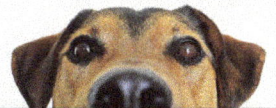

Signs of Significant Blood Loss in Dogs:

- **Pale or white gums:**
    - This is often a sign of reduced blood in circulation.
        - While there are other causes for pale gums, those always require a veterinary assessment.
- **Weakness or lethargy:** Lack of energy is a common symptom.
- **Rapid or shallow breathing:** Dogs may breathe quickly or irregularly due to reduced red blood cells and oxygen carrying capacity.
- **Cold extremities:** There may be a drop in body temperature due to poor circulation.
- **Behavioral changes:** Your dog may become unusually quiet, disoriented, or less responsive.
- **Dilated pupils:** Enlarged pupils may indicate a lack of blood flow to the eyes.
- **Seizures:** In severe cases, significant blood loss can lead to seizures.

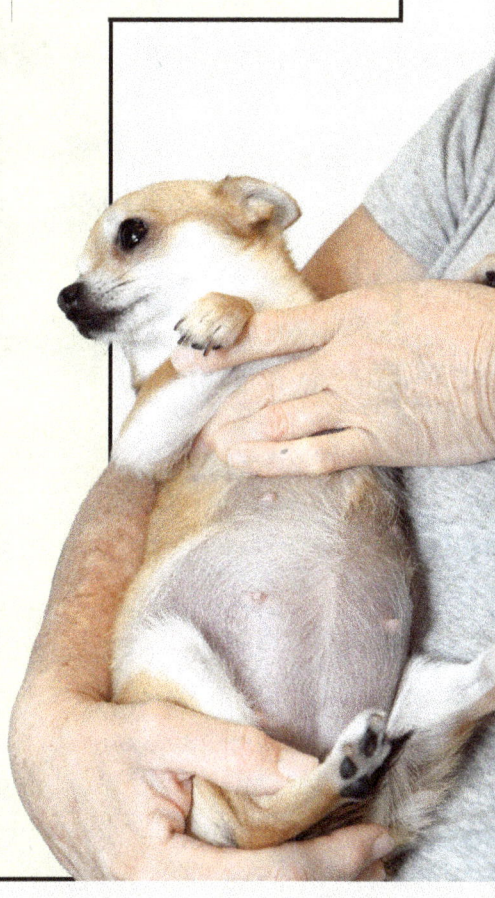

When to Seek Veterinary Care?

External Bleeding: If you are unable to stop the bleeding after applying pressure or if the injury is large or deep, contact your veterinarian immediately.

Internal Bleeding: If your dog shows any of the signs of significant blood loss, such as pale gums, weakness, or rapid breathing, seek emergency veterinary care immediately. Internal bleeding is serious and can worsen quickly without intervention.

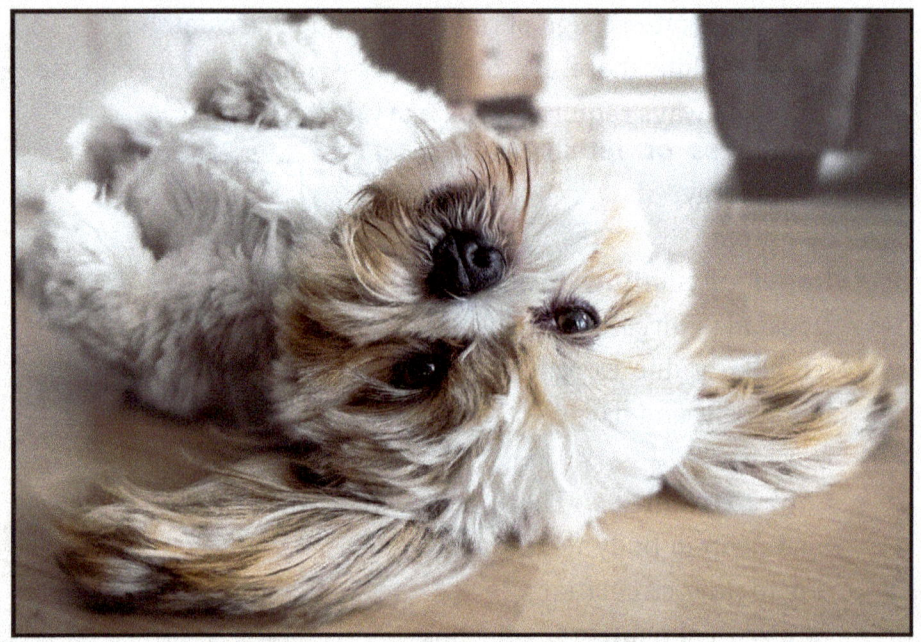

SUMMARY:

Bleeding, whether external or internal, requires quick attention. External bleeding can often be controlled with pressure, but larger wounds or those that don't stop bleeding need veterinary care. Internal bleeding is harder to detect, but signs like pale gums, weakness, and rapid breathing should prompt immediate veterinary attention. Act quickly to ensure your dog's safety and well-being.

OVERVIEW
- Minor trauma
- Major trauma
- When to respond

Possible Emergency

TRAUMA
(PHYSICAL INJURY)

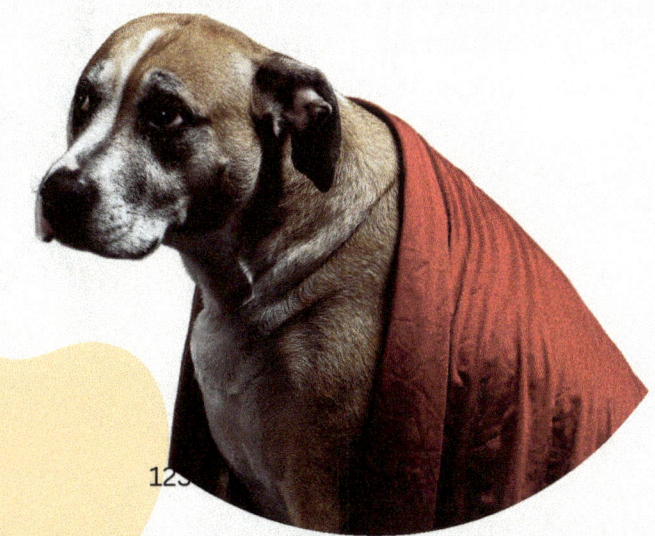

Trauma can happen in many forms, and the level of concern varies depending on the type, severity, and the dog's response. Both minor and major trauma can cause significant issues, some of which may not be immediately apparent. Here's how to assess and respond to different types of trauma:

Minor Trauma

Minor injuries are common and may result from incidents like falling from furniture, tripping, or missing a step.

While these situations might not seem serious - especially in larger dogs - there are key signs to watch for that may indicate a more significant issue. Those include:

1. loss of consciousness
2. inability to use a limb
3. sudden changes in behavior
4. pain or sensitivity to touch

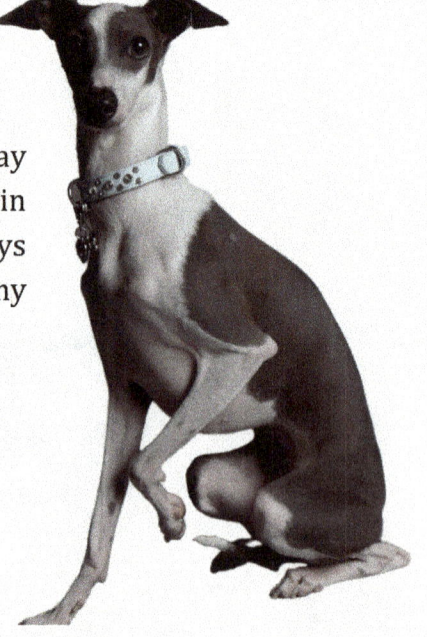

Keep in mind that small dogs may sustain severe injuries, even in situations that seem minor. Always be cautious and aware of any unusual behavior after an injury.

Major Trauma

Major trauma involves more significant injuries, often resulting from falls from elevated heights, falls down flights of stairs, or being struck by a vehicle.

While these incidents may not always have visible damage, they can cause serious injuries, such as broken bones, internal injuries, or head trauma.

Watch for the following signs:
1. Pale gums (a sign of blood loss or shock)
2. Weakness or lethargy
3. Poor responsiveness
4. Loss of consciousness
5. Changes in breathing patterns (e.g., rapid or shallow breathing)

In these cases, internal injuries or bleeding may not be visible, but they are often life-threatening. Immediate veterinary attention is crucial for the proper diagnosis and treatment.

When to Seek Veterinary Care?

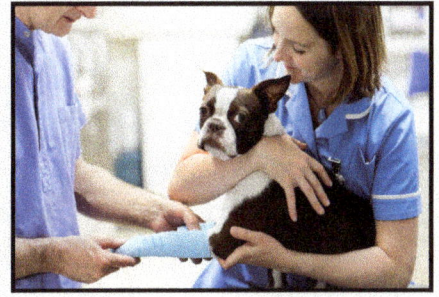

Any trauma leading to pain, discomfort, or visible injury should be assessed by a veterinarian. If your dog shows any of the signs above, especially after a significant injury, you should seek immediate veterinary care. Even if the injury seems minor, it's always better to be evaluated by a veterinarian.

SUMMARY:

Trauma can range from minor to severe, and its seriousness depends on the type, severity, and your dog's response. Minor trauma, like falls from furniture, may not seem serious but can still cause concern if your dog shows signs like loss of consciousness or limping. Major trauma, such as falls from heights or vehicle accidents, can cause severe internal injuries that may not be visible. Watch for signs like pale gums, weakness, or abnormal breathing. In any case of trauma, acting quickly and seeking veterinary care is essential.

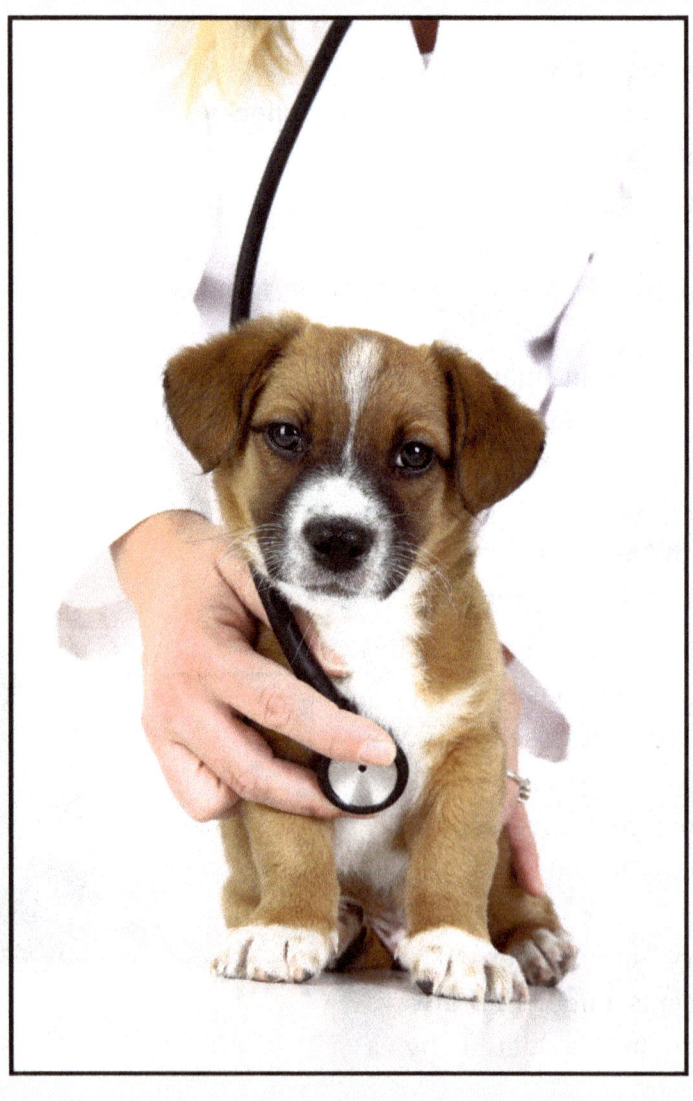

OVERVIEW

- Distended abdomen
- Accompanying signs of concern

Possible Emergency

BLOATED/ DISTENDED ABDOMEN

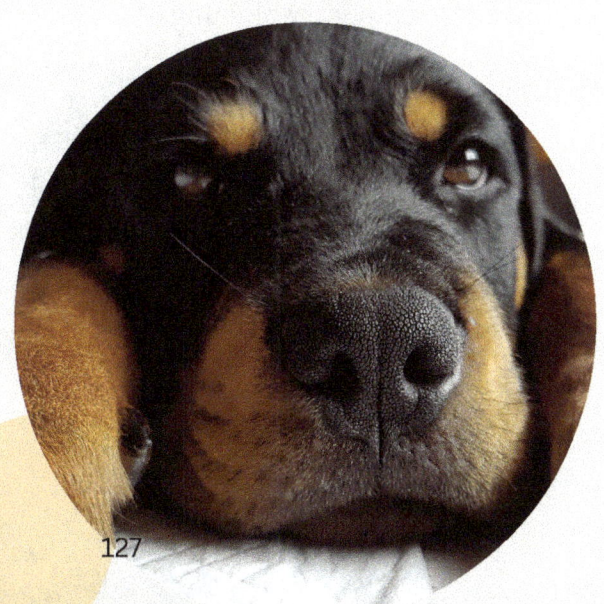

A distended or bloated belly can indicate anything from a benign condition to a life-threatening emergency. The urgency of the situation depends on the accompanying signs and symptoms. Below is an overview of possible causes and signs to notice.

Common Causes of a Distended Belly
LESS SERIOUS

- Parasites: Severe infestations of intestinal worms, particularly in puppies, can lead to an enlarged belly.
- Pregnancy: In female dogs, pregnancy causes abdominal enlargement as the puppies grow.
- Organ Enlargement: Conditions like an enlarged spleen or liver can cause noticeable changes in the abdomen.
- Tumors: Abdominal masses can alter the shape and size of the belly.
- Cushing's Disease: This condition, due to excess cortisol, weakens abdominal muscles and leads to a "pot-bellied" appearance.
- Obesity/Weight Gain: Excess fat can also cause the belly to appear distended.
- Gas Accumulation: Excess gas in the gastrointestinal tract can lead to temporary bloating.

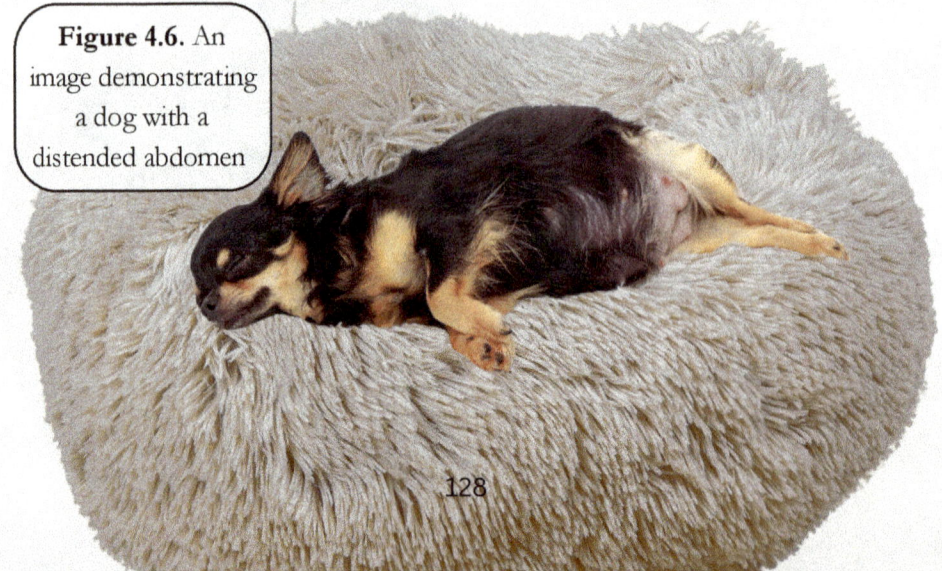

Figure 4.6. An image demonstrating a dog with a distended abdomen

Common Causes of a Distended Belly
MORE SERIOUS

- <u>Bloat</u> (GDV or Gastric Dilatation Volvulus): This is a serious and life-threatening condition where the stomach fills with gas and twists.
- <u>Food Bloat</u>: This happens when a dog overeats and the stomach becomes overfull with food and gas. This is less serious than a GDV but often requires emergency assessment.
- <u>Fluid Accumulation</u>: This occurs due to various causes such as liver disease, heart failure, infections, or hemoabdomen (bleeding in the abdomen).
- <u>Intestinal Obstruction:</u> A blockage in the intestines can lead to swelling, pain, and abdominal distention.
- <u>Infections or Inflammatory Conditions</u>: Conditions like pancreatitis or peritonitis cause abdominal swelling due to inflammation or fluid buildup.

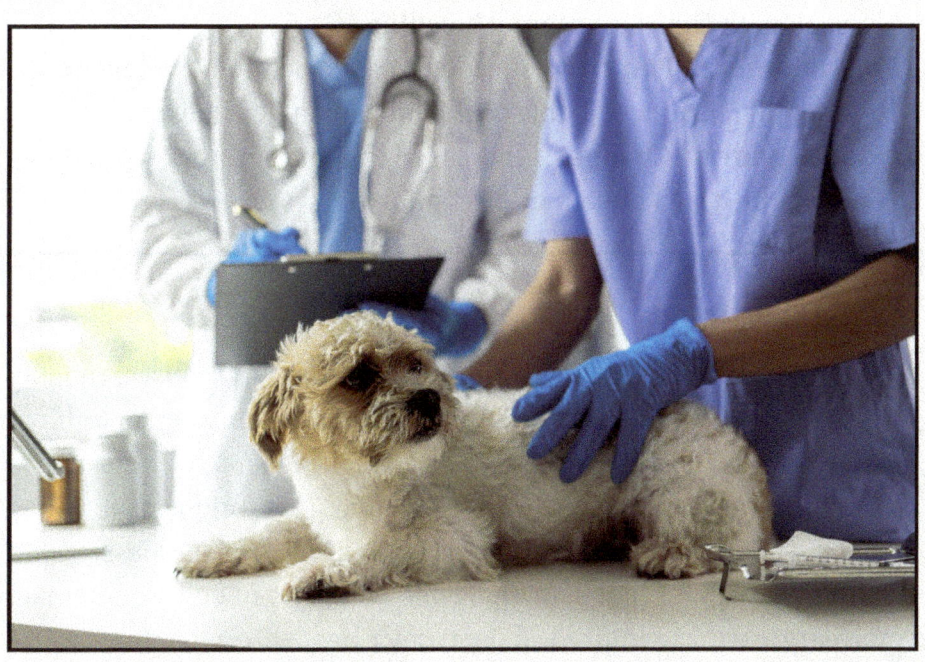

When to Seek Veterinary Care?

To help determine the severity of the abdominal distension, look out for the following signs, which indicate the need for immediate veterinary care:

- **Unsuccessful Vomiting**: If your dog attempts to vomit but cannot bring anything up, it could indicate a blockage or GDV.
- **Restlessness:** Anxiety, pacing, or difficulty finding a comfortable position may signal discomfort or pain.
- **Rapid Breathing:** Increased breathing rate can indicate pain, distress, or reduced blood circulation.
- **Excessive Drooling:** This can be a sign of nausea or severe discomfort.
- **Weakness or Lethargy:** A sudden drop in energy or inability to stand can indicate a serious underlying issue.
- **Pale Gums:** This suggests reduced blood circulation, often seen with shock or internal bleeding.
- **Abdominal Pain:** If your dog reacts painfully when their abdomen is touched, this could indicate internal distress.
- **Behavioral Changes:** Increased agitation or restlessness could be a sign of pain or discomfort.

SUMMARY:

A bloated or distended belly in dogs can have many causes, ranging from harmless weight gain to life-threatening conditions like bloat (GDV). Recognizing the difference between a benign cause and a serious emergency depends on accompanying symptoms. If your dog exhibits signs such as unsuccessful vomiting, restlessness, rapid breathing, or abdominal pain alongside an enlarged belly, immediate veterinary care is required. It is always best to err on the side of caution and consult a veterinarian.

OVERVIEW

- Potential causes
- Steps to follow if collapse is seen

SKILLS TOOLKIT

- Collapse response steps

True emergency!

COLLAPSE

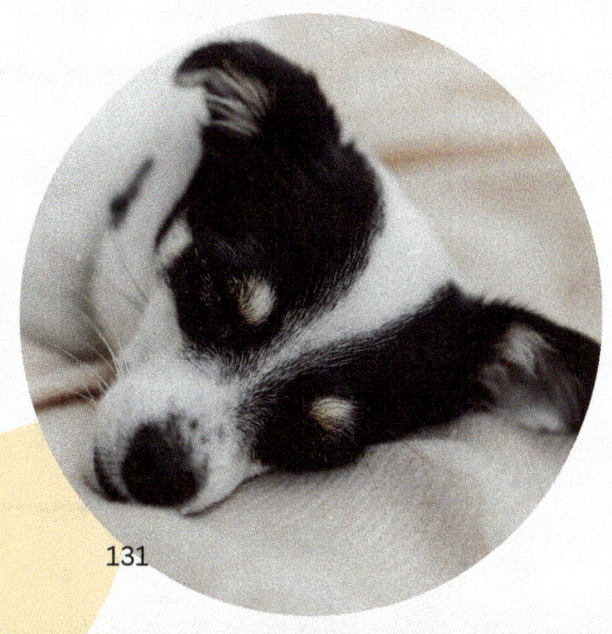

If your dog suddenly collapses or loses consciousness, it could signal a serious medical emergency. Rapid recognition and response can be crucial in preventing further complications. Below, we break down the potential causes, signs to watch for, and steps to take if your dog collapses.

Potential Causes of Sudden Collapse

- **Cardiac Issues (Heart Disease or Arrhythmias)**: Heart conditions can cause sudden collapse due to poor blood flow to the brain, often resulting in fainting episodes called <u>syncope.</u>
- **Stroke or Vascular Accident**: Disrupted blood flow to the brain, often caused by a blood clot, can lead to sudden unconsciousness.
- **Trauma:** Falls, accidents, or physical injuries can lead to internal bleeding, traumatic brain injury, neurological damage, or shock.
- **Seizures**: Seizures can cause collapse, followed by confusion or disorientation (see the seizure chapter for more information).
- **Hypoglycemia** (Low Blood Sugar): Dogs, especially small breeds or those with pre-existing health conditions, can experience fainting or weakness from low blood sugar.
- **Heatstroke:** Overheating, often during hot weather or after vigorous exercise, can cause collapse.

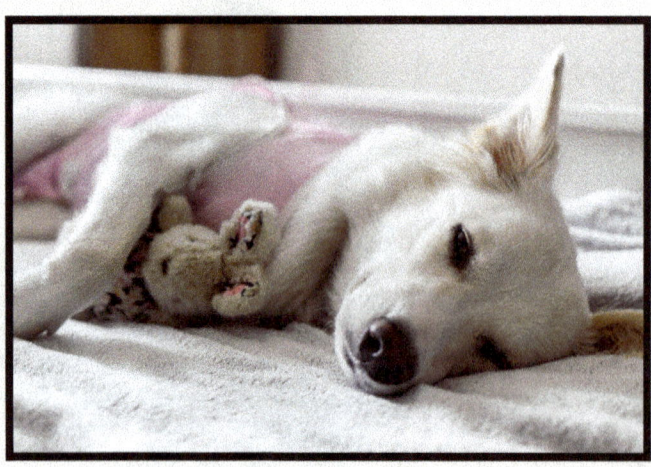

What to Do if Your Dog Collapses

- **Check for Responsiveness:** Gently call your dog's name or tap them lightly to see if they respond.
- **Assess Breathing:** Check to see if your dog is breathing normally - and note the rate and effort. If you suspect difficulty breathing, refer to the respiratory distress section.
- **Look for Injuries:** If there is any chance your dog fell or suffered an impact, inspect for visible injuries, particularly fractures or internal trauma.
- **Prepare for Transport:** If your dog is unresponsive, keep them comfortable and minimize movement unless absolutely necessary. If transport is needed, support their body to prevent additional harm.
- **Contact a Veterinarian:** Call ahead and inform your veterinarian of the emergency, so they can be prepared for immediate evaluation upon your arrival.

When to Seek Veterinary Care

Collapse episodes generally require immediate veterinary attention. An emergency veterinary visit is required.

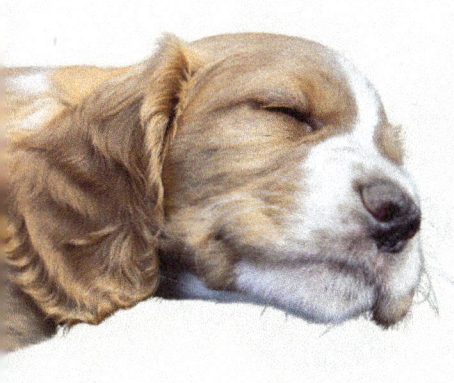

SUMMARY:

Sudden collapse or unconsciousness in dogs can indicate serious underlying issues such as heart conditions, trauma, or vascular accidents. Recognizing the signs, such as pre-collapse behavior, changes in posture, or abnormal breathing, can help guide your response. If your dog collapses, it's crucial to do what you can to keep them safe before contacting a veterinarian.

OVERVIEW

- Common causes
- Signs to notice
- Response

SKILLS TOOLKIT

- Responding to a dog in pain
- BONUS: Pain scales/ scores

True emergency!

SEVERE PAIN/ DIFFICULTY MOVING

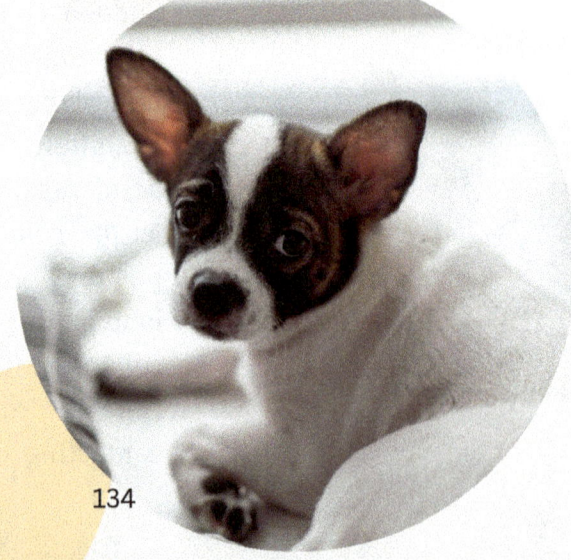

If your dog is showing signs of severe pain or is unable to move normally, it may indicate a serious injury or medical condition. Recognizing the cause and responding appropriately is critical to ensuring your pet receives the right care.

Common Causes of Severe Pain or Difficulty Moving

- **Injuries:** Fractures, sprains, or strains from accidents or rough play can cause significant pain.
- **Joint Issues:** Conditions like arthritis or hip dysplasia can lead to chronic discomfort and difficulty moving.
- **Internal Conditions:** Problems like pancreatitis, abdominal trauma, or organ rupture can cause severe internal pain.
- **Neurological Issues:** Spinal injuries or intervertebral disc disease can result in difficulty moving or severe pain.

Signs of Pain

Not all dogs show pain in the same way. Below are some common ways by which dogs demonstrate pain:

- **Vocalization:** yelping, whining, or crying when moving or being touched
- **Posture:** holding limbs in an unusual position or exhibiting a hunched back
- **Limping:** favoring one leg or avoiding putting weight on a limb
- **Restlessness**: pacing, inability to find a comfortable position, or excessive panting
- **Changes in Behavior:** withdrawal, aggression when touched, or loss of appetite

What to do If Your Dog is in Pain

- **Limit Movement:** Keep your dog still to prevent further injury. Provide a comfortable resting space.
- **Assess for Injuries:**
  - Gently examine limbs, joints, and abdomen for swelling, heat, or tenderness.
  - If your dog reacts to touch, avoid applying pressure to that area.
- **Monitor Symptoms:** Keep track of changes in behavior, eating, and drinking. Note the duration of pain and any new symptoms.
- **Call your vet or an emergency clinic** to describe your dog's symptoms and any potential injuries.
  - Follow their advice on whether to bring your dog in for an evaluation.
- **Prepare for Transport:**
  - If necessary, use a padded crate or blanket to support your dog during transport.
  - Be careful when lifting or moving to prevent worsening injuries.

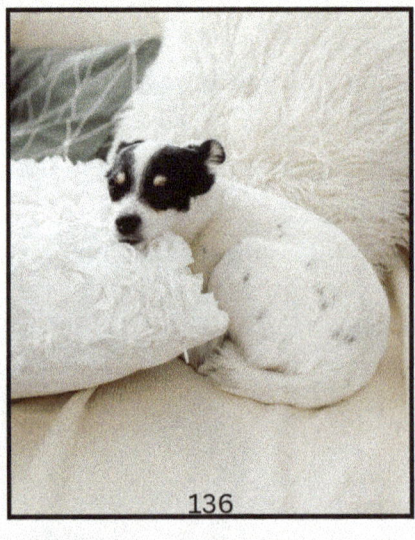

Understanding Pain Scores in Dogs

A pain score is a numerical system used to assess and quantify the level of pain an animal is experiencing. It helps veterinarians and pet owners communicate about pain levels effectively, guide treatment decisions, and evaluate treatment success.

Why Pain Scores Matter
- Dogs can't verbally express their pain.
- Individual dogs may behave differently at the same pain level.
- Pain scales use behavioral and physical signs to categorize pain levels.

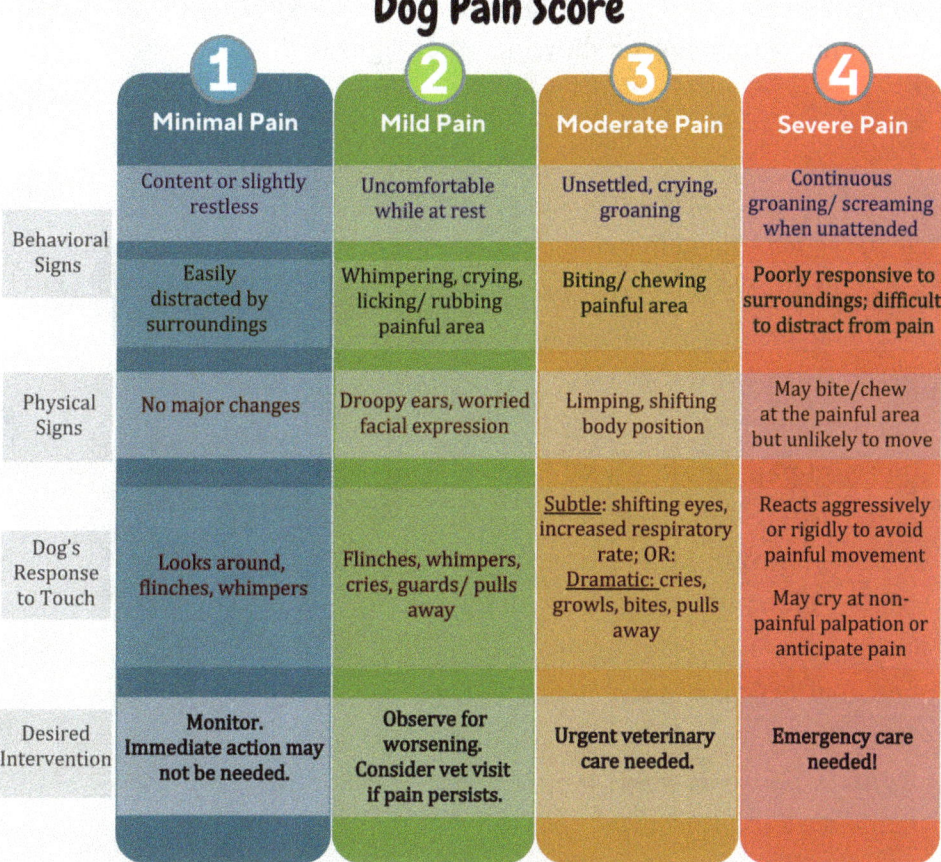

Figure 4.7: Summary of the Colorado State University Canine Acute Pain Scale

When to Seek Veterinary Care?

Seek veterinary care:
- when your dog is in severe pain (Score 3 or 4) or shows signs of significant distress.
- when there are visible injuries.
- when your dog is unable to move or bear weight on a limb, which may suggest fractures, sprains, or neurological issues.
- when there is a behavioral change like aggression when touched, withdrawal, or loss of appetite.
- when the pain persists for more than a few hours or worsens despite comfort measures.

Immediate veterinary attention is necessary if your dog is in severe pain, unable to move, or showing other signs of distress.

SUMMARY:

Severe pain or difficulty moving in dogs can result from various causes, including injuries, joint issues, or internal conditions. Recognizing signs like vocalization, limping, or changes in behavior is crucial for identifying pain.

Immediate veterinary care is often required if your dog is in severe pain or shows signs of trauma. By using pain scales, limiting movement, and following veterinary advice, you can help ensure your dog's recovery and well-being. Always trust your instincts. If your dog is in pain, seek veterinary care without delay.

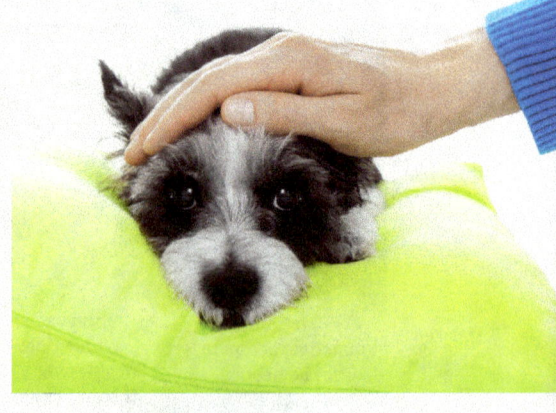

SUBTLE SYMPTOMS YOU SHOULDN'T IGNORE

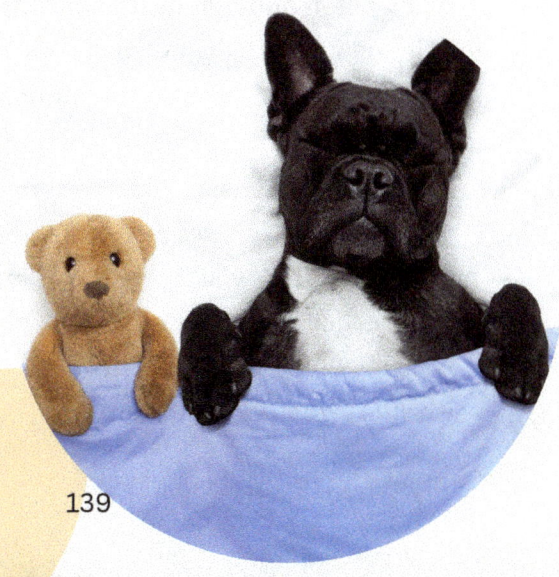

Sometimes, emergencies aren't immediately obvious. Your dog may not be bleeding or having a seizure, but certain subtle symptoms still warrant attention.

Watch for these signs:

- **Unusual Behavior:** If your typically friendly and playful dog suddenly becomes agitated, aggressive, or unusually withdrawn, it may indicate an underlying health issue. Pain or illness often manifests as behavioral changes, so take note and consider seeking help.

- **Excessive Thirst or Urination:** While dogs may drink more after exercise, sudden excessive thirst or urination could signal conditions like kidney disease, diabetes, or urinary tract infections.

- **Coughing or Gagging:** Persistent coughing, gagging, or retching can indicate a respiratory infection, kennel cough, or even heart disease. If these symptoms don't resolve quickly or worsen, consult your veterinarian.

- **Abnormal Gait or Difficulty Walking:** If your dog limps, drags a leg, or has trouble standing or walking, it may be due to joint, muscle, or neurological issues. Don't assume it will improve on its own; prompt care can prevent long-term problems.

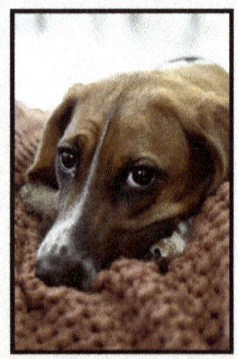

These signs do not necessarily require an immediate visit with an emergency veterinarian. However, they do warrant a call to your veterinarian!

WHAT TO DO IN AN EMERGENCY

If you suspect an emergency, here's what you can do:

- <u>Stay Calm:</u> Your dog can sense your anxiety. Remaining calm will help you make clearer decisions and keep your dog relaxed.

- <u>Contact Your Vet or an Emergency Clinic:</u> Clearly describe the signs and ask for guidance. Some situations may require immediate action, while others may involve basic first aid instructions over the phone.

- <u>Follow Instructions Precisely</u>: Following the recommendations of the veterinarian can make all the difference in how your dog responds to care.

CONCLUSION

This chapter provided a basic overview about signs that may indicate a true emergency, as well as signs that indicate the likely need for priority care with a vet. Also introduced were various skills that can be used to help observe and monitor your pet, so you can feel more secure in assessing for possible concerns. This knowledge will further assist you when communicating with the vet and will ensure everyone is on the same page.

In many situations, it's better to be safe than sorry. If you're ever uncertain about whether your dog's condition is an emergency, don't hesitate to reach out to your veterinarian or an emergency clinic. Quick action and appropriate care can make a significant difference in your dog's well-being. As a pet owner, trust your instincts. Your dog relies on you to make the right call in times of need. Remember, your vigilance and prompt response could save your dog's life.

Chapter 5

PREVENTING EMERGENCIES

While emergencies are often unavoidable, there's much you can do to prevent them from happening in the first place. By pet-proofing your home, practicing safe outdoor activities, recognizing potential hazards in your dog's diet and surroundings, and ensuring routine vet care, you can dramatically reduce the risk of emergencies.

Chapter Highlights

1. Pet Proofing Your Home

2. Safe Outdoor Practices

3. Routine Checkups

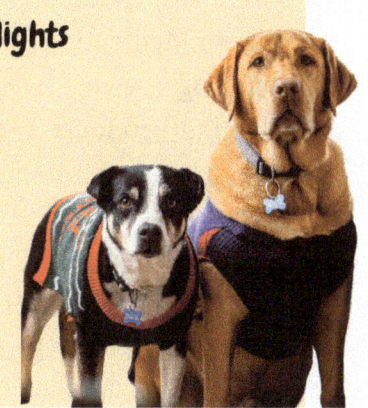

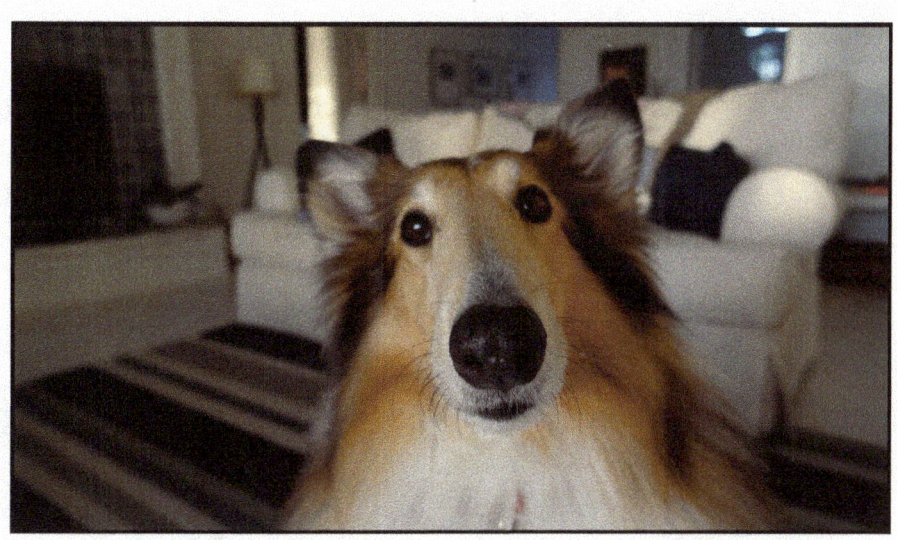

Pet-Proofing Your Home

Just as you would baby-proof a home for a child, it's essential to pet-proof your living space to keep your dog safe.

- **Keep Toxic Foods and Substances Out of Reach**
    - <u>Harmful Foods:</u> Keep foods that may be harmful to dogs out of reach (i.e., chocolate, grapes, and raisins).
    - <u>Human Medications:</u> Never leave pills or medications within your dog's reach.
    - <u>Cleaning Products and Chemicals</u>: Store household cleaners up high or in cabinets with childproof locks.
    - <u>Plants:</u> Some plants (like sago palm, azalea, and foxglove) are toxic to dogs, so keep them out of the house or yard.
- **Prevent Burns or Injuries:**
    - Protect your dog from the <u>fireplace, stovetop, or candles</u>. Burns from hot surfaces or open flames can be serious injuries.
    - Ensure your dog doesn't have access to <u>hot water heaters</u> or <u>radiators</u>.
- **Protect from Sharp Objects/ Edges:**
    - Items like <u>scissors, knives</u>, and even <u>sharp-edged furniture</u> can cause cuts and wounds. Keep these stored safely out of your pet's reach. Also, check your yard for sharp objects like broken glass or metal that could injure your dog while playing outside.
- **Electrical Safety:**
    - Dogs are naturally curious and may chew on <u>wires or cords</u>. Cover up outlets and use cord protectors to avoid electric shocks.
- **Secure Trash and Food:**
    - Use <u>pet-proof trash cans</u> and avoid leaving food on counters where it's easily accessible.

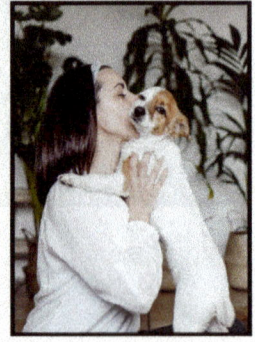

Safe Outdoor Practices

When it comes to outdoor activities, there are several ways you can ensure your dog stays safe while exploring the world around them.

- **Supervise Outdoor Play**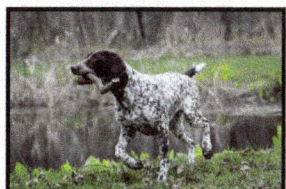
    - While playing outside, keep a close eye on your dog to prevent accidents.
- **Fenced Yards and Leashes**
    - Make sure your backyard is securely fenced to prevent escapes.
    - On walks, always use a leash to prevent your dog from running off or getting into dangerous situations (like traffic, other aggressive dogs, or wild animals).
    - Leashes should ideally be six feet long or less. Injuries are seen with use of retractable leashes.
- **Safe Play Areas**
    - Avoid public parks or areas with little to no supervision where hazards can be hidden (e.g., glass or sharp rocks).
- **Temperature Awareness**
    - Always be mindful of the weather. Avoid walking your dog during the hottest parts of the day. Also be mindful of the ground temperature. Sidewalks or asphalt can become dangerously hot for their paws.
- **Swimming Safety**
    - If you live near water, make sure your dog is comfortable and safe around water. Not all dogs are natural swimmers. Consider a dog life vest if your dog is not a proficient swimmer, especially around rivers, lakes, or oceans.
- **Ticks and Fleas**
    - Keep your dog on preventative medications and regularly check for ticks, especially after hikes or trips to wooded areas. Ticks can transmit diseases like Lyme disease, so immediate removal is essential.

Routine Checkups

Routine visits to the vet are an essential part of keeping your dog healthy and preventing emergencies. Many serious conditions, like heart disease, diabetes, kidney disease, and more, can be caught early with regular check-ups.

- **Annual Vet Check-Ups:**
    - Regular vet visits help catch potential health issues early. Even if your dog seems perfectly healthy, an annual wellness exam can spot hidden issues that could develop into major problems.
    - Some veterinarians recommend visits every six months as a dog ages.
- **Vaccinations and Parasite Prevention:**
    - Keep your dog up to date on their vaccinations, especially Rabies.
    - Regular flea, tick, and heartworm prevention is also crucial and should be given year-round in many places.
- **Dental Care:**
    - Dental disease is often overlooked but can lead to painful infections and even organ damage. Regular brushing, dental chews, and professional cleanings can help keep your dog's teeth healthy.
- **Spaying/Neutering:**
    - Spaying or neutering your dog not only helps prevent unwanted litters but also reduces the risk of certain cancers and health complications later in life.
- **Monitoring Weight and Diet:**
    - Keeping your dog at a healthy weight can help reduce the odds of certain emergencies. Ensure you're feeding a balanced diet and engaging in regular exercise to maintain their physical condition.

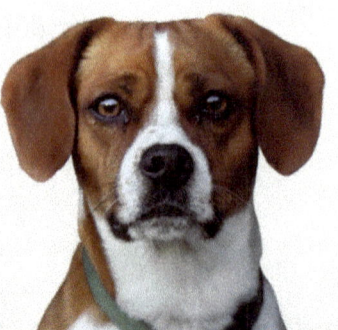

Chapter 6

YOUR EMERGENCY TOOLKIT RECAP

Figure 6.1

BREATHING RATE EVALUATION:
Resting Respiratory Rate (RRR):
Used to monitor your dog's breathing rate over time

Process
- Watch the chest rise and fall
- Count the number of breaths in 6 seconds
- Multiply by 10
  - This is your breaths/minute

Normal: Fewer than 40 breaths per minute

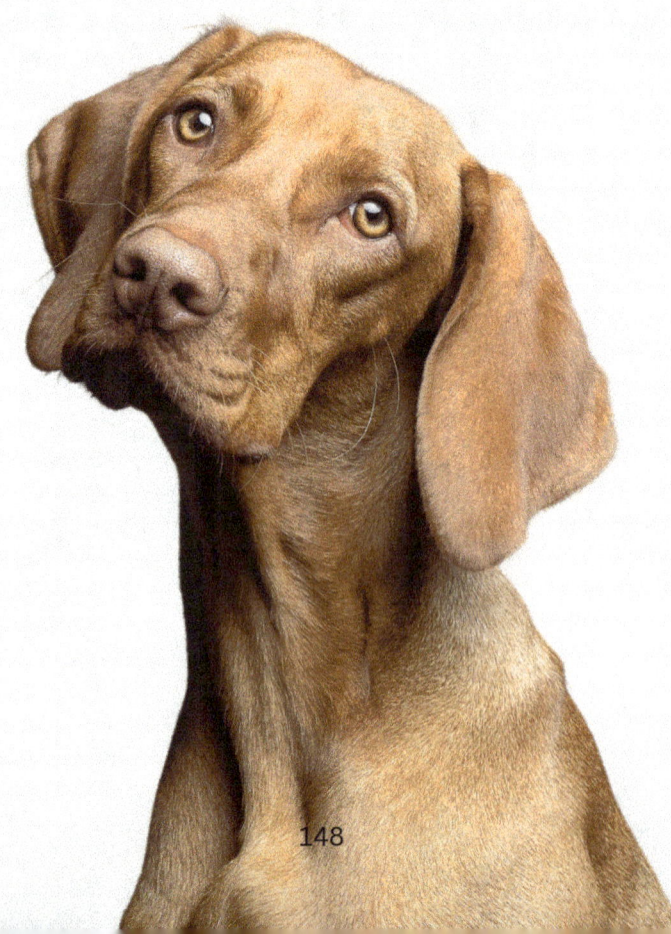

DEHYDRATION EVALUATION:

Gum Moisture Assessment

Lift your dog's lips to examine the gums.
Swipe your fingers across the gums to assess moisture.

Normal: Moist gums
Abnormal: Tacky gums, which may indicate dehydration

Eye Assessment

Evaluate the eyes for appearance and positioning.

Normal: Bright, clear, moist eyes that sit comfortably in their socket
Abnormal: Dull or sunken eyes

Skin Tenting

Gently pinch the skin on the back of your dog's neck or between the shoulder blades using your thumb and forefinger. Release the skin and observe how quickly it returns to normal.

Normal: Skin returns to normal position in <1 second
Mild Dehydration: Skin remains tented for 1-2 seconds
Moderate/Severe Dehydration: Skin tenting for >2seconds

Capillary Refill Time (CRT)

Expose your dog's gums. Gently press on the gum area until it is white (<1 second) and then release.

Normal: Color returns in <2 seconds
Abnormal: Prolonged response of >2seconds

Figure 6.2

If your dog is experiencing pain, consider the following measures:

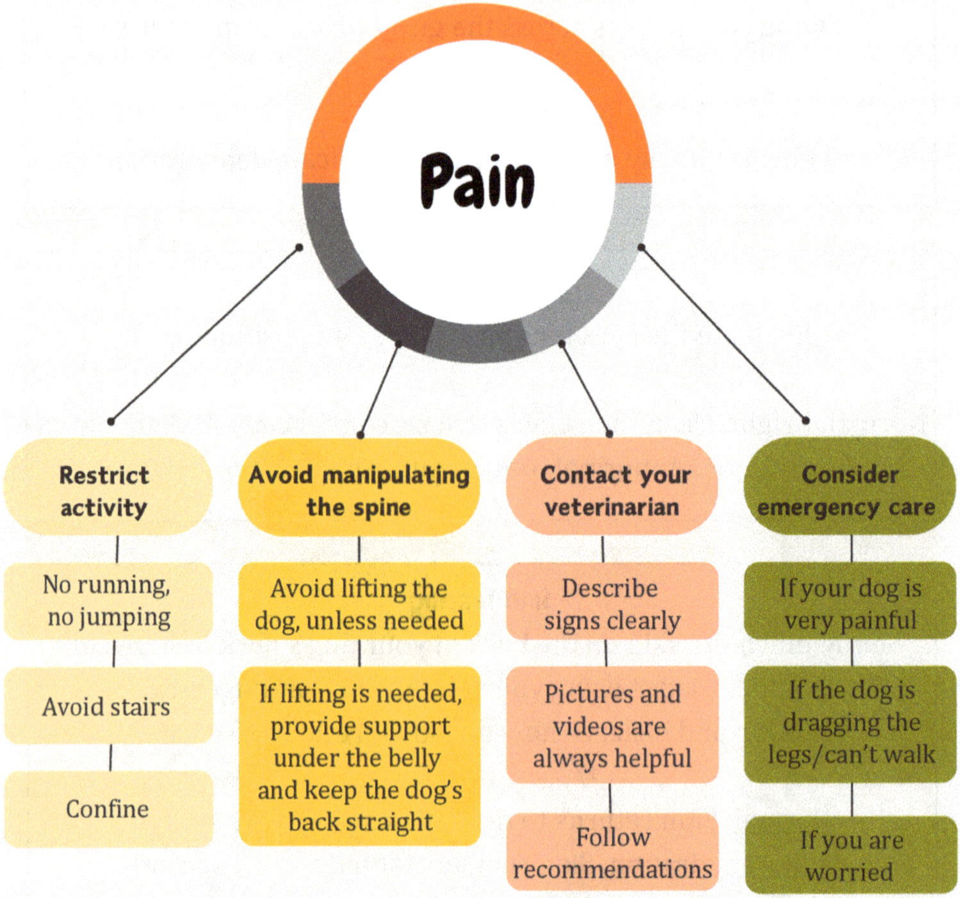

Pain

Restrict activity
- No running, no jumping
- Avoid stairs
- Confine

Avoid manipulating the spine
- Avoid lifting the dog, unless needed
- If lifting is needed, provide support under the belly and keep the dog's back straight

Contact your veterinarian
- Describe signs clearly
- Pictures and videos are always helpful
- Follow recommendations

Consider emergency care
- If your dog is very painful
- If the dog is dragging the legs/can't walk
- If you are worried

Figure 6.3: Pain chart

These steps are provided as a guide and are not in a specific order. If veterinary care is needed, please prioritize seeking professional help and don't feel the need to complete all steps first.

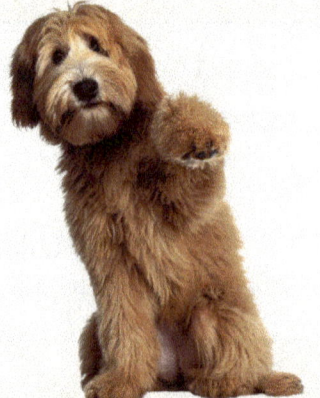

If your dog is overheated, consider the following measures:

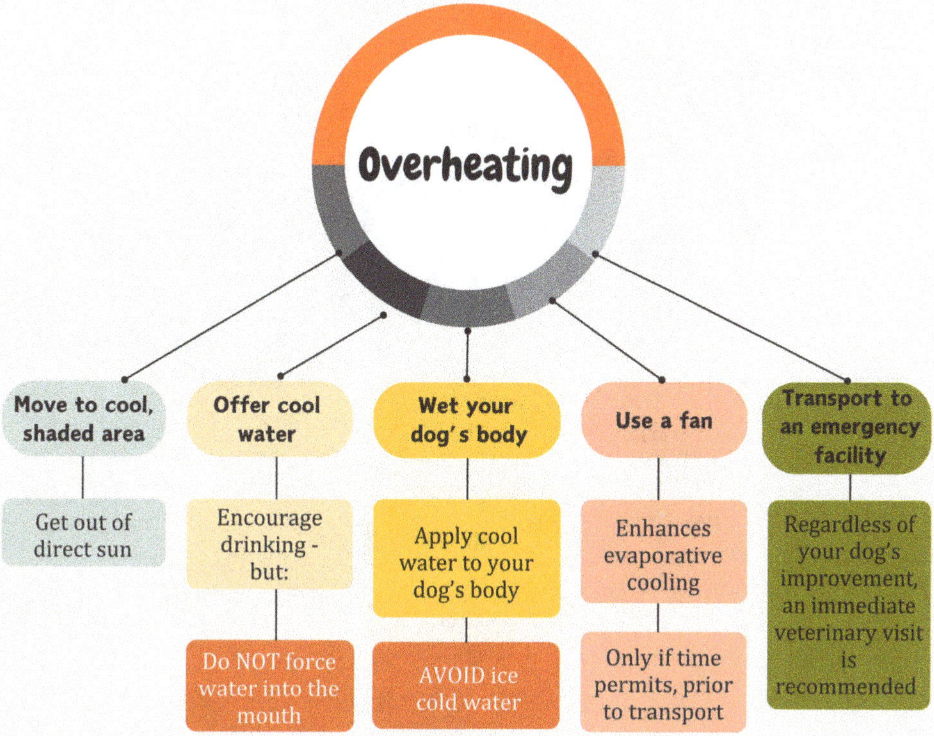

```
                        Overheating
     ┌──────────┬──────────┬──────────┬──────────┐
Move to cool,  Offer cool  Wet your   Use a fan  Transport to
shaded area      water    dog's body             an emergency
                                                    facility

Get outof     Encourage   Apply cool  Enhances   Regardless of
direct sun     drinking -  water to   evaporative your dog's
               but:       your dog's  cooling    improvement,
                          body                   an immediate
                                                 veterinary visit
              Do NOT force AVOID ice  Only if time is
              water into the cold water permits, prior recommended
              mouth                    to transport
```

Figure 6.4: Overheating response chart

These steps are provided as a guide and are not in a specific order. If veterinary care is needed, please prioritize seeking professional help and don't feel the need to complete all steps first.

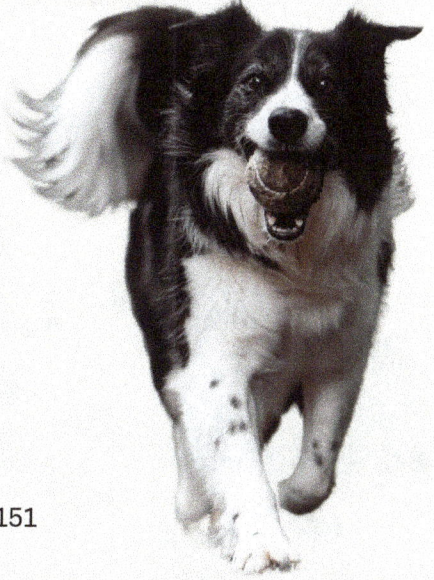

In case of an allergic reaction, consider the following measures:

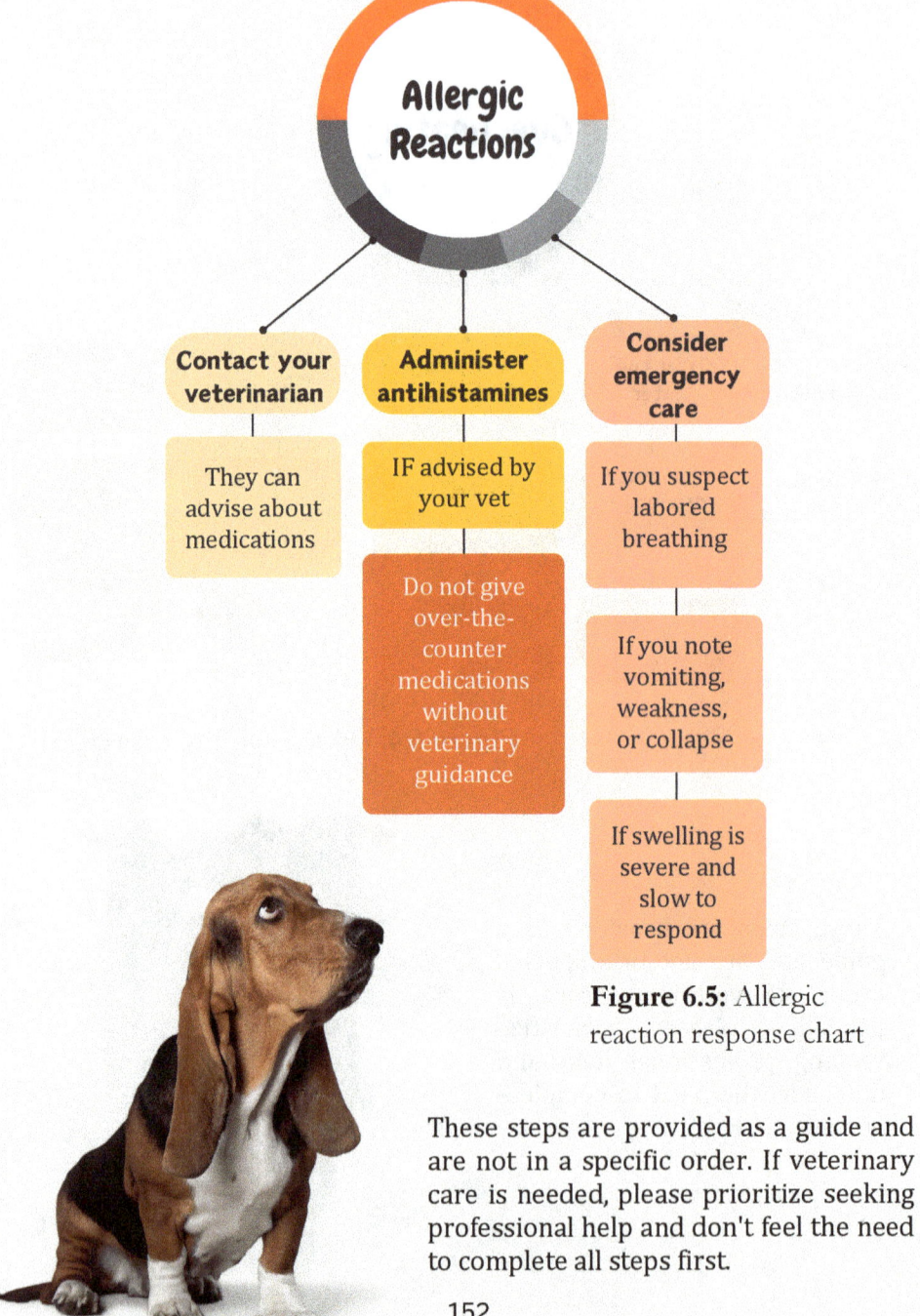

Figure 6.5: Allergic reaction response chart

These steps are provided as a guide and are not in a specific order. If veterinary care is needed, please prioritize seeking professional help and don't feel the need to complete all steps first.

If your dog is experiencing breathing difficulties, consider the following measures:

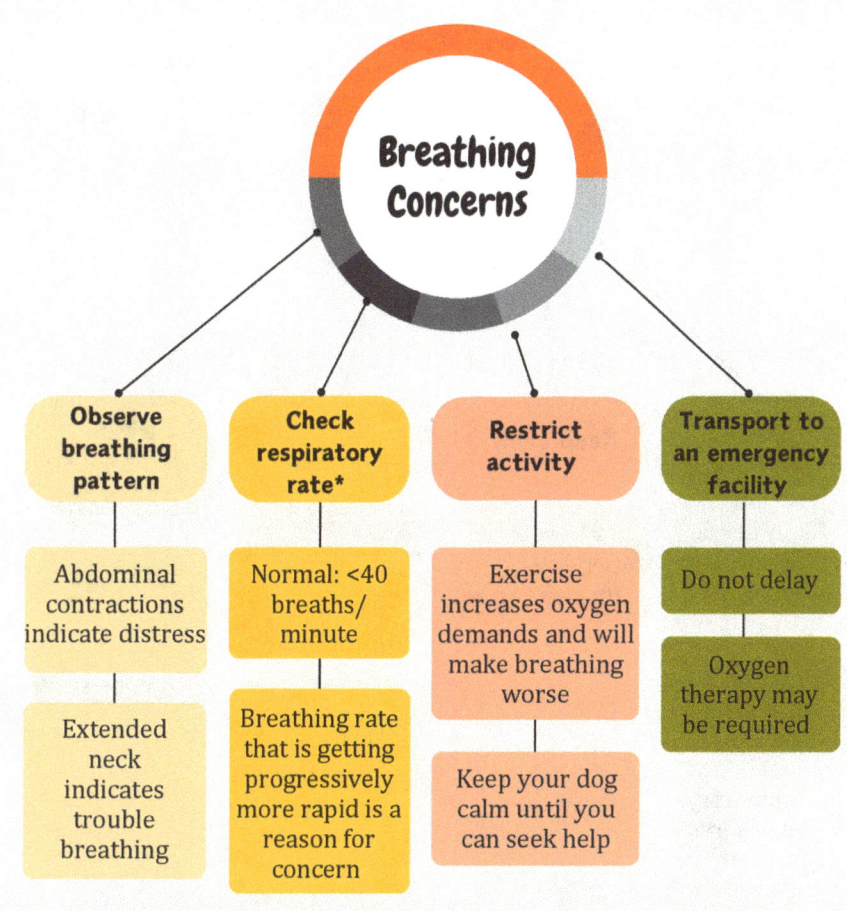

Figure 6.6: Breathing concerns response chart

These steps are provided as a guide and are not in a specific order. If veterinary care is needed, please prioritize seeking professional help and don't feel the need to complete all steps first.

*Refer to the Resting Respiratory Rate section for a tutorial on how to check respiratory rate.

If your dog has a bite wound, consider the following measures:

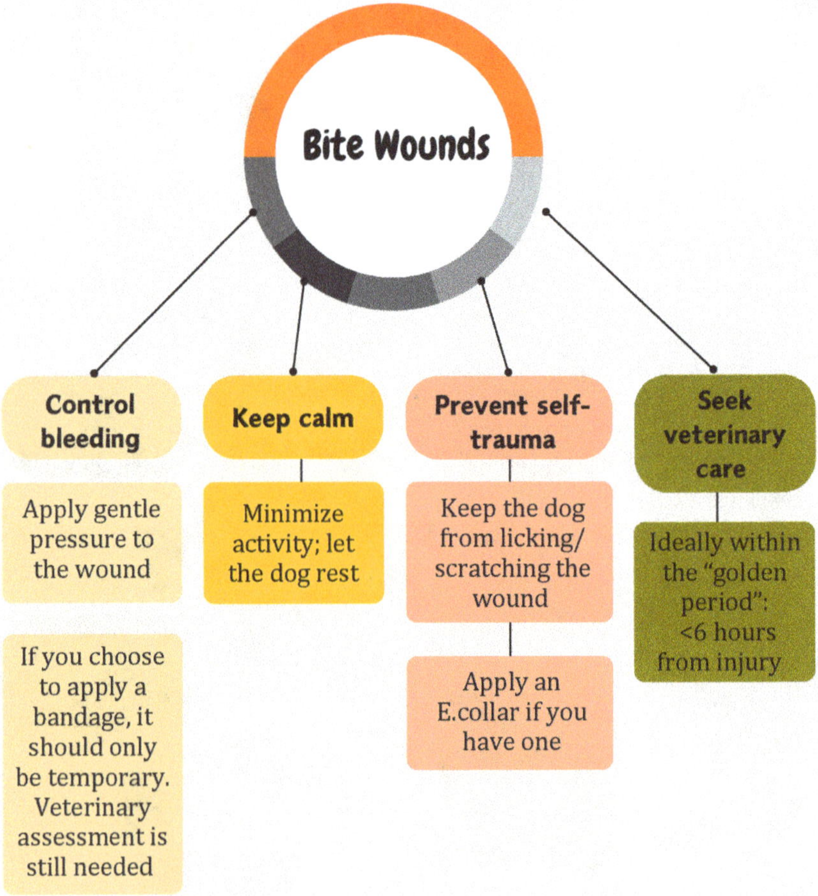

Bite Wounds

Control bleeding
- Apply gentle pressure to the wound
- If you choose to apply a bandage, it should only be temporary. Veterinary assessment is still needed

Keep calm
- Minimize activity; let the dog rest

Prevent self-trauma
- Keep the dog from licking/scratching the wound
- Apply an E.collar if you have one

Seek veterinary care
- Ideally within the "golden period": <6 hours from injury

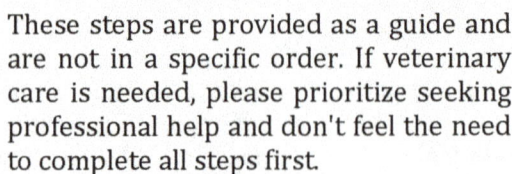

Figure 6.7: Bite wounds response chart

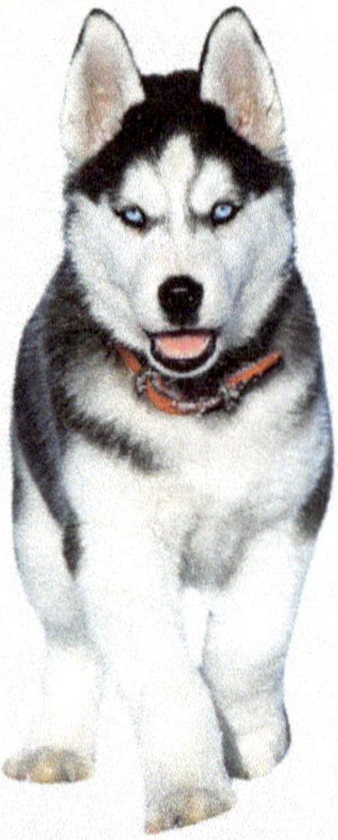

These steps are provided as a guide and are not in a specific order. If veterinary care is needed, please prioritize seeking professional help and don't feel the need to complete all steps first.

If your dog has collapsed, consider the following measures.

Most dogs recover quickly from a collapse episode. However, if your dog remains unresponsive, safely transport your dog to a veterinarian immediately.

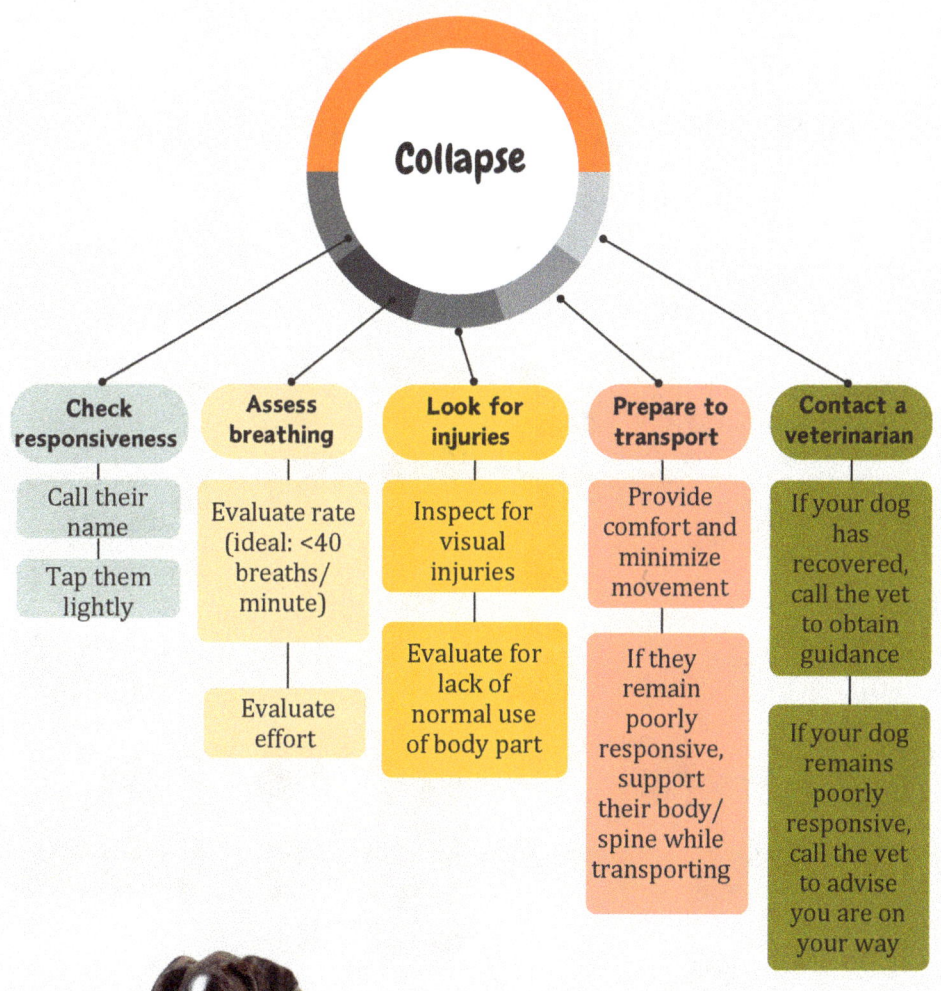

Figure 6.8: Collapse response chart

These steps are provided as a guide and are not in a specific order. If veterinary care is needed, please prioritize seeking professional help and don't feel the need to complete all steps first.

If your dog has a bleeding toenail, consider the following measures:

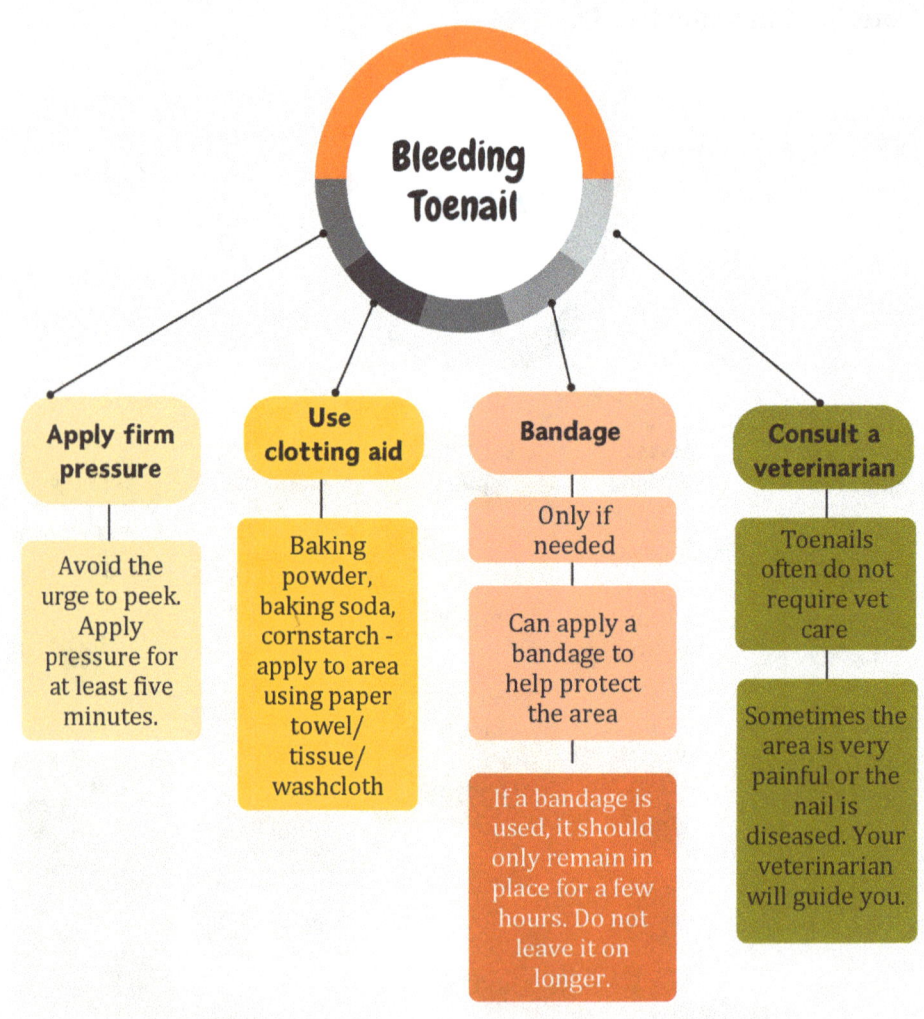

Figure 6.9: Bleeding toenail response chart

If your dog has a seizure, follow the flow chart to assess urgency

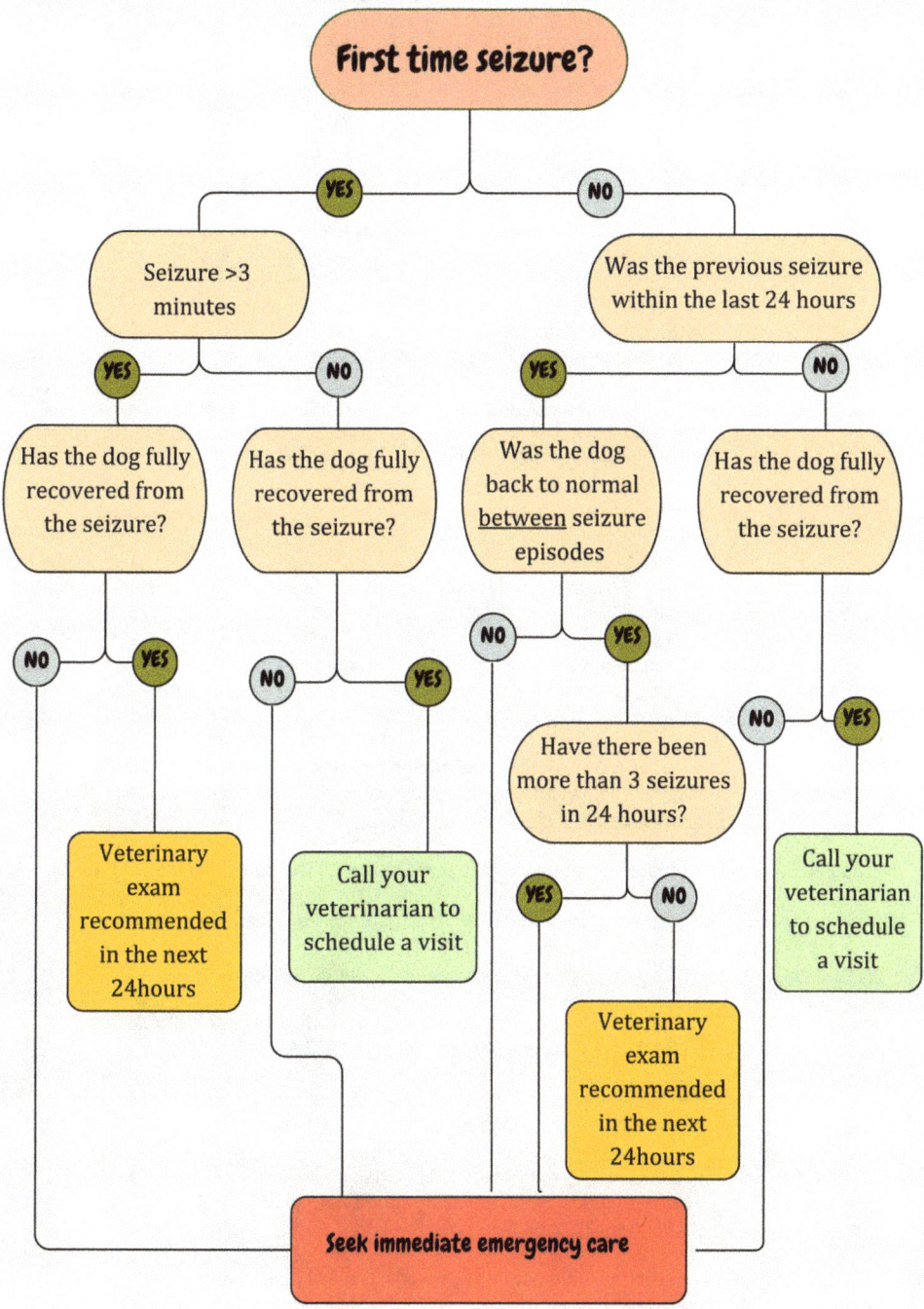

Figure 6.10: Seizure response chart

REFERENCES
& ADDITIONAL RESOURCES

ASPCA Animal Poison Control Center. (n.d.). Pet poisoning and toxicology. American Society for the Prevention of Cruelty to Animals. Retrieved January 7, 2025, from https://www.aspca.org/pet-care/animal-poison-control

Barton, P. R., & Jeffery, N. D. (2013). "Traumatic Injuries in Dogs: A Review of Common Clinical Presentations and Management Strategies." Veterinary Surgery, 42(7), 846-856.

Boudrieau, R. J., & Richardson, D. C. (2002). Management of bite wounds in dogs: Clinical presentation and treatment protocols. Veterinary Clinics of North America: Small Animal Practice, 32(5), 1093-1107. https://doi.org/10.1016/S0195-5616(02)00042-9

Dudley, R. M., et al. (2010). Canine bite wounds: Diagnosis, treatment, and complications. Journal of the American Veterinary Medical Association (JAVMA), 236(4), 453-458. https://doi.org/10.2460/javma.236.4.453

Fossum, T. W. (2018). "Heat Stress and Heatstroke in Dogs." In Small Animal Surgery (5th ed.). Elsevier.

Fossum, T. W. (2018). "Surgical Treatment of Gastric Dilatation-Volvulus in Dogs." In Small Animal Surgery (5th ed.). Elsevier.

Fossum, T. W., & Van der Linde, L. (2006). Management of foreign body ingestion in dogs: A review of 100 cases. Veterinary Clinics of North America: Small Animal Practice, 36(4), 1005-1016. https://doi.org/10.1016/j.cvsm.2006.02.004

Goddard, A. A., & Sullivan, M. P. (2008). A review of canine bite wounds and their clinical management in veterinary practice. Journal of Veterinary Emergency and Critical Care, 18(2), 120-126. https://doi.org/10.1111/j.1476-4431.2008.00290.x

Halliwell, R. E. (2006). "Breed Predispositions to Disease in Dogs." The Veterinary Journal, 172(1), 1-8.

Hellyer, P. W., Uhrig, S. R., & Robinson, N. G. (2006). The Colorado Pain Scale. Colorado State University Veterinary Teaching Hospital. https://vetmedbiosci.colostate.edu/vth/services/anesthesia/animal-pain-scales/

Johnstone, S. F. F., et al. (2013). Risk factors for splenic rupture in dogs: 93 cases (2001–2011). Veterinary Surgery, 42(6), 713-721. https://doi.org/10.1111/j.1532-950X.2013.01055.x

Lam, R., & Smith, P. (2015). "Canine Intervertebral Disc Disease: Pathophysiology, Diagnosis, and Treatment." The Veterinary Journal, 204(3), 225-231.

Le, D. D. M., et al. (2012). Clinical features and outcome of hemorrhagic abdominal effusion in dogs. Veterinary Clinics of North America: Small Animal Practice, 42(6), 1055-1065. https://doi.org/10.1016/j.cvsm.2012.08.005

Licht, D. J., et al. (2014). Hereditary epilepsy in dog breeds: Genetic predispositions and disease management. Veterinary Medicine and Surgery, 42(7), 1305-1313. https://doi.org/10.1111/j.1476-4431.2014.01184.x

Liu, J., & Petty, J. P. (2016). "Trauma in Dogs: Clinical Management of the Acute Trauma Patient." Veterinary Clinics of North America: Small Animal Practice, 46(5), 927-939.

Liptak, J. M., & Glickman, L. T. (2004). Foreign body ingestion in dogs: Diagnosis, treatment, and breed-specific considerations. Journal of Veterinary Internal Medicine, 18(3), 263-268. https://doi.org/10.1892/0891-6640(2004)018<0263:FBIDT>2.0.CO;2

Lunardi, A. L., & Buhl, L. L. (2018). "Canine Atopic Dermatitis: A Review of the Role of Genetics in Predisposition and Clinical Expression." Veterinary Dermatology, 29(3), 174-182.

MacNeill, J. A., et al. (2014). Breed-related risks for hemangiosarcoma in dogs. Veterinary Pathology, 51(6), 1132-1141. https://doi.org/10.1177/0305735614532499

Mawby, D. I., et al. (2012). Seizure disorders in dogs: Breed and genetic considerations. Journal of the American Veterinary Medical Association (JAVMA), 241(3), 336-341. https://doi.org/10.2460/javma.241.3.336

McKee, W. M., & Paterson, D. (2017). "Trauma and its Effects on the Canine Spine and Musculoskeletal System." Journal of Small Animal Practice, 58(9), 521-527.

McLaren, C., Null, J., & Quinn, J. (2005). Heat stress from enclosed vehicles: Moderate ambient temperatures cause significant temperature rise in enclosed vehicles. Pediatrics, 116(1), e109–e112. https://doi.org/10.1542/peds.2004-2368

Milan, M., & Thomas, M. L. (2017). "Heatstroke in Dogs: Prevention, Diagnosis, and Treatment." Veterinary Clinics of North America: Small Animal Practice, 47(4), 689-698.

Patsolas, M., & McKee, W. M. (2019). "Intervertebral Disc Disease in Dogs: A Review of Diagnosis and Surgical Treatment." Journal of Small Animal Practice, 60(6), 348-355.

Ricciardi, C. P. M., et al. (2011). Hemangiosarcoma of the spleen in dogs: 25-year review of cases and clinical outcomes. Journal of Veterinary Internal Medicine, 25(4), 527-534.

Reimer, J. M., & Schneider, R. A. (2012). "Canine Trauma and Its Impact on Orthopedic Injuries." Veterinary Orthopedics and Traumatology Journal, 25(3), 204-212.

Schertel, E. R., & Glickman, L. T. (2010). "Breed Predispositions to Gastric Dilatation-Volvulus (GDV) in Dogs." Journal of Veterinary Internal Medicine, 24(1), 88-95.

Scott, D. W., Miller, W. H., & Griffin, C. E. (2001). Müller and Kirk's Small Animal Dermatology (6th ed.). Saunders.

Smith, P. M., & Johnson, S. C. (2014). "Heatstroke in Dogs: Pathophysiology, Risk Factors, and Management." Journal of Veterinary Emergency and Critical Care, 24(1), 7-15.

Toll, D., et al. (2011). Epidemiology and management of congestive heart failure in dogs. Veterinary Clinics of North America: Small Animal Practice, 41(6), 1219-1235. https://doi.org/10.1016/j.cvsm.2011.07.006

Dr. Gal Chivvis

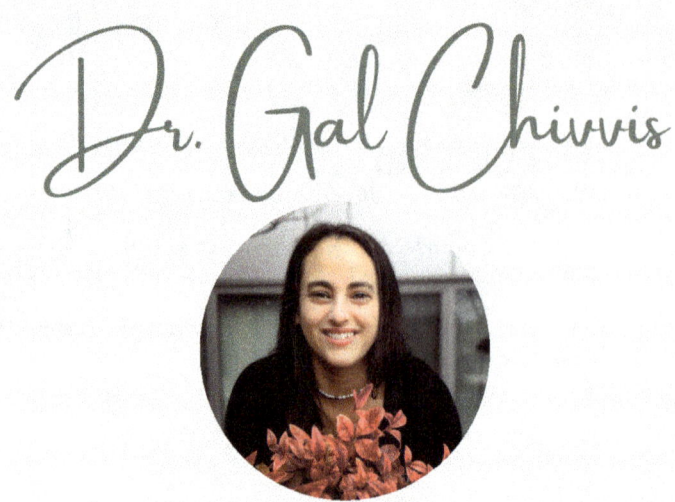

Dr. Gal Chivvis is an emergency veterinarian with over a decade of experience and the founder of Critter Care Collective—"One Team, One Goal: Collaborative Pet Care." She is committed to making pet health information accessible and engaging for all pet owners.

Dr. Chivvis has authored multiple books, including a children's picture book series, activity books, ABC books, and adult coloring books, all designed to educate, entertain, and relieve stress. She also shares valuable pet health resources on her website, www.crittercarecollective.com.

With a passion for collaboration, Dr. Chivvis works to bridge the gap between veterinary professionals and pet owners, hoping this book empowers you to navigate pet health emergencies with confidence.

- ✉ CritterCareCollective@gmail.com
- 🌐 www.CritterCareCollective.com
- 🌐 www.TheDVMAuthor.com
- 📷 @crittercarecrew
- 📷 @TheDVMAuthor

Thank You!

Thank you for choosing this guide to help you care for your dog during life's unexpected moments. I designed this resource to offer clear, practical advice when you need it most. I firmly believe that the best care for our pets comes from collaboration between informed pet owners and dedicated veterinary professionals. I hope you found the book valuable.

Download free copies of the forms from this book by scanning the QR code or visiting www.crittercarecollective.com.

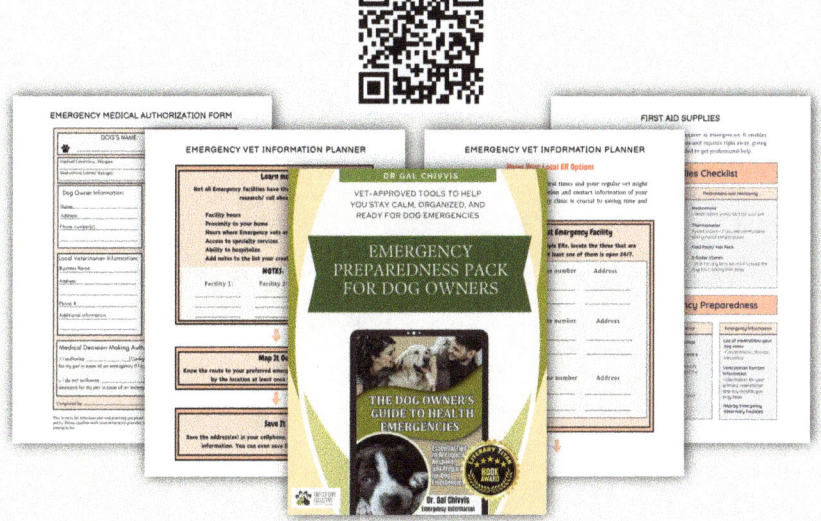

In addition to educational materials for adults, I create engaging resources for children, including activity books, picture books, and relaxing coloring books. Explore more of these on my website or Amazon.

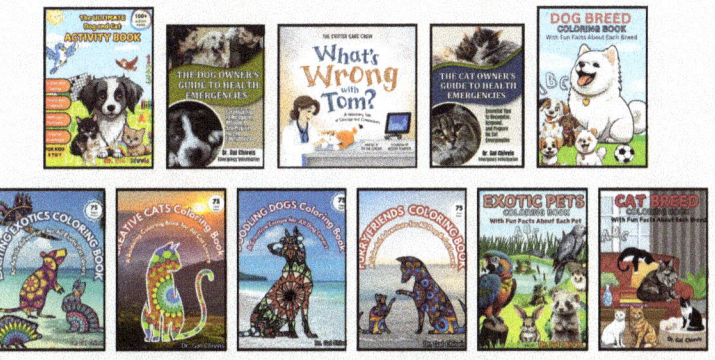

www.ingramcontent.com/pod-product-compliance
Lightning Source LLC
Chambersburg PA
CBHW060503030426
42337CB00015B/1717